Guide to Healthy
Fast-Food
Eating

Hope S. Warshaw
MMSc, RD, CDE, BC-ADM

American Diabetes Association.
Cure • Care • Commitment®

Director, Book Publishing, John Fedor; *Managing Editor,* Abe Ogden; *Acquisitions Editor, Consumer Books,* Robert Anthony; *Editor,* Rebecca Lanning; *Production Manager,* Melissa Sprott; *Composition,* ADA; *Cover Design,* Koncept, Inc.; *Printer,* United Graphics, Inc.

Printed in the United States of America
1 3 5 7 9 10 8 6 4 2

ADA titles may be purchased for business or promotional use or for special sales. To purchase this book in large quantities, or for custom editions of this book with your logo, contact Lee Romano Sequeira, Special Sales & Promotions, at the address below, or at LRomano@diabetes.org or 703-299-2046.

American Diabetes Association
1701 North Beauregard Street
Alexandria, Virginia 22311

Library of Congress Cataloging-in-Publication Data

Warshaw, Hope S., 1954–
  Guide to healthy fast-food eating / Hope S. Warshaw.
     p. cm.
  Includes bibliographical references and index.
  ISBN-13: 978-1-58040-270-5 (alk. paper)
  1. Diabetes—Diet therapy. 2. Diabetics—Nutrition. 3. Fast food restaurants—United States. I. Title.

  RC662.W3152 2006
  616.4'620654—dc22

                              2006031395

To people with diabetes who, on a daily basis, strive to manage their blood glucose and prevent diabetes complications. May the knowledge and information you gain from this book help you stay healthy and complication free.

— HSW

Contents

Preface

This compact and easy-to-carry *Guide to Healthy Fast-Food Eating* contains two main sections. In the first, you'll find out how to eat healthily with diabetes and learn about the pitfalls of restaurant eating—lots of fat, big portions, and way too much sodium. You'll also gather the skills and strategies you need to make healthier food choices in all types of restaurants.

In section 2, you'll find a baker's dozen (13) of the top fast-food restaurant chains across the nation. With more than 100,000 locations worldwide, these popular fast-food restaurants are the ones most people frequent most often. They are also the restaurants for which the most nutrition information is now available.

In our fast-paced, convenience-focused world, most people will continue to choose fast-food restaurant meals. You'll eat these at the restaurant, in your office, at home, or at the ball field. It's just a way of getting the job of eating done today. With some skills and strategies under your belt and nutrition facts in hand, you can reach your goals to eat healthily; keep your blood glucose, blood lipids, and blood pressure on target; and stay well for many years to come.

I encourage you to keep asking for nutrition information from any restaurant you eat in and to support federal and state legislation requiring restaurant chains to provide this information. If enough of us keep asking, eventually they'll give us the facts.

In health,
Hope S. Warshaw, MMSc, RD, CDE, BC-ADM

Acknowledgments

This book would have been impossible to create without the cooperation and assistance from many people at the corporate headquarters of many restaurant chains and the willingness of many other chains to provide their nutrition information on their Web sites. On behalf of the people with diabetes who will use and benefit from the information in the pages ahead, I am indebted to these restaurant chains. They set an example of public responsibility for the rest of the chain restaurant industry.

No book is completed by just the author alone. In this case, I am grateful to Paula Payne, RD, who assisted with the development of the nutrient database and other aspects of the book. Thanks also to all those at ADA who supported this effort: Rebecca Lanning, Editor; Melissa Sprott, Production Manager; Robert Anthony, Acquisitions Editor; Abe Ogden, Managing Editor; and John Fedor, Director, Book Publishing.

A last word of thanks goes to my professional colleagues, who consistently lend their ears and ideas. They continue to be a source of inspiration and encouragement.

Section 1:
Healthy Restaurant Eating

Today's Diabetes Eating Goals

During the 1990s diabetes eating goals underwent a minor revolution. In fact, the phrase "diabetic diet" is now a misnomer. No such diet exists. No longer must you ax sugary foods and sweets from your list of acceptable foods. Now you can savor the taste of a few slices of pizza at the popular chain pizza shops or cruise to the drive-thru for a hamburger, a small order of fries, and a garden salad when time is not on your side.

The current diabetes eating goals encourage you to eat healthfully and to do what it takes to keep your blood glucose levels in the normal range as much as possible. These goals also recommend that you keep your blood lipids (fats) and blood pressure on target, because carefully managing all three of these blood levels is what will keep you healthy over the years.

Your diabetes plan should work around your needs and lifestyle and not vice versa. Your health care providers have many more tools today to help you formulate a diabetes care plan that works for you. The end goal, of course, is to prevent or slow down long-term diabetes complications, such as eye, heart, and kidney problems.

Diabetes Eating Goals in a Nutshell

In 2006, the American Diabetes Association (ADA) put forth four key nutrition goals.

1. To the extent that you are able, achieve and maintain your diabetes ABCs:

   A is for A1C. Keep your blood glucose levels in the normal range or as close to normal as possible.
   A1C: <7%
   Fasting and before meals
      blood glucose: 90–130 mg/dl
   Blood glucose 2 hours
      after the start of a meal: <180 mg/dl

   B is for blood pressure. Keep your blood pressure <130/80 mmHg to help prevent heart disease and strokes.

   C is for cholesterol. Aim for healthy blood lipid levels—LDL cholesterol (bad), HDL cholesterol (good), and triglycerides—to help prevent heart disease and strokes.
   LDL: <100 mg/dl
   HDL: >40 mg/dl (men), >50 mg/dl (women)
   Triglycerides: <150 mg/dl

2. Try to prevent, or at least delay, the long-term and chronic complications of diabetes by making appropriate lifestyle changes and choosing healthy foods.

3. Consult with your health care providers and diabetes educators to find an eating plan that works for you. This eating plan should take into account your food preferences and your cultural practices as well as your willingness to make changes in your current eating habits.

4. Continue to enjoy eating and avoid limiting your food choices while also achieving and maintaining good health.

These are the nutrition goals. But what foods should you eat to reach these goals? Here are tips to focus on:

- Eat more (six or more servings) grains, beans, and starchy vegetables each day. Make three of these servings whole grains.
- Eat more fruits and vegetables. Strive for 2 1/2 cups of vegetables and 2 cups of fruit a day.
- Include two to three servings of fat-free or low-fat dairy foods each day—milk, yogurt, and cheese—within your calorie allotment. They provide calcium and other important nutrients.
- Eat a small to moderate amount of meat and other protein foods. Two 3-oz servings each day are enough for most people. Not only does eating less meat help you eat less protein, it also makes it easier for you to eat less total fat, saturated fat, and cholesterol.
- Go light on fats and oils. Limit oils that are high in saturated fat and trans fat, such as coconut and palm oils. Limit partially hydrogenated fats in commercially prepared foods and fried restaurant foods, which may contain trans fats. Limiting fried foods is a good way to limit trans fats when you eat in restaurants.
- Limit foods that are high in cholesterol (such as whole-milk dairy foods, egg yolks, and organ meats).
- Enjoy small amounts of sugary foods and sweets just once in a while. If you have some pounds to shed or your blood glucose or blood fats are not in your target range, eat sweets more sparingly. If you're on the slim side, you can splurge on sweets a bit more often if you choose to.
- Drink no more than one alcoholic drink a day if you are a woman and two drinks a day if you are a man.

One drink is defined as 1 1/2 oz of hard liquor (a shot), 12 oz of beer, or 5 oz of wine.

Everybody Sings the Same Song

Take note: The ADA recommendations for healthy eating echo the way all Americans are encouraged to eat—even Americans at risk for heart disease or some cancers. Whether it's the American Heart Association, the American Cancer Society, or the U.S. government, every organization is singing this same nutrition song.

This means that as a person with diabetes, your nutrition goals are in sync with the nutrition goals of your family members, friends, and neighbors. That's not to say that healthy eating is simple or that you won't sometimes feel like a fish swimming upstream because so many Americans chow down on unhealthy foods—and large portions of them. Remember, it's not easy to eat healthfully. And that is particularly true when it comes to restaurant foods.

How Much Should You Eat?

Base what you eat each day on the servings and types of foods noted above. Eat these foods in reasonable amounts. When and how much you eat should match your lifestyle and schedule. Another critical element is to determine which foods and times for meals and snacks work best to help you manage your blood glucose, blood lipids, and blood pressure. The best choices you make to care for your diabetes are those that help you feel good day to day and help prevent or slow down the development of diabetes problems.

No set number of calories is right for everyone with diabetes. The number of calories you need depends on many factors. A few of them are your height, your age, your current weight and whether you want to lose weight or are at a healthy weight, whether you have a hard or easy time losing weight, your daily activity level, and the type of physical activity you normally do.

Always have a meal plan and method of meal planning that fit you and your lifestyle. To develop a meal plan and healthy eating goals that you are comfortable with and that factor in your individual needs, work with a registered dietitian (RD) with diabetes expertise, such as a certified diabetes educator (CDE). A dietitian can help you learn how to work almost any food into a healthy eating plan or to solve your meal planning dilemmas. For instance, maybe you travel several days a week and eat all your meals in restaurants. (To find diabetes education programs near you, see "Help Is Nearby," on pages 8 and 9.)

Several books published by the ADA on food, nutrition, and meal planning give more in-depth information about how much and what you should eat.

Myriad Approaches to Meal Planning

Once you know what and how much to eat, you and a dietitian can zero in on a meal planning approach that fits your needs. If you want a simple approach, for example, then the diabetes food pyramid may be best for you. Or if you are willing to check your blood glucose several times a day and do some math, then you might opt for carbohydrate counting.

You may be familiar with the diabetes exchange system as the way some people with diabetes learn to plan meals. The ADA and the American Dietetic Association's *Exchange Lists for Meal Planning* dates back to 1950. The exchange system has been revised a number of times. The last revision was in 2003. Today, the exchange system is no longer the only way to do diabetes meal planning. You can use a food group approach, carbohydrate gram counting, fat gram counting, or the point system, to name a few options. The right meal planning approach for you is the one that you can learn and put to work. One approach might be right for you when you first develop diabetes, and then down the road another approach may work best as you change the way you manage your diabetes.

Any Meal Planning Approach Works in Restaurants

No matter which meal planning approach you use, you can take advantage of the information in this book. If you opt for the exchange system or the diabetes food pyramid, use the food servings or exchanges noted in the charts. If you do carbohydrate counting, then the grams of carbohydrate and grams of dietary fiber are where you want to focus. Zero in on the calories and fat if fat gram counting is part of your meal planning method.

Help Is Nearby

Whether you have just found out you have diabetes or you have been doing the diabetes balancing act for years, you can always learn more. Get to know a diabetes educator. A diabetes educator can help you tailor your diabetes management plan and offer tips for dealing with diabetes. The following resources are a good start to link you up with quality diabetes care:

- To find a Recognized Diabetes Education Program (a teaching program approved by the American Diabetes Association) near you, call 1-800-DIABETES (1-800-342-2383), look at ADA's Internet home page, www.diabetes.org, or go straight to www.diabetes.org/education/eduprogram.asp.
- To find diabetes educators (who may be dietitians, nurses, pharmacists, counselors, or other health professionals) near you, call the American Association of Diabetes Educators (AADE) toll-free at 1-800-TEAMUP4 (1-800-832-6874) or go to AADE's Internet site at www.aadenet.org and go to "Find an Educator."

Here's more good news: It may now be easier for you to take advantage of the services of a diabetes educator or diabetes education program (known in Medicare parlance as Diabetes Self-Management Training) as well as a dietitian. Medicare now covers diabetes education and nutrition counseling (known as Medical Nutrition Therapy) for diabetes in many new settings for those with Medicare Part B. Also, in nearly all states across the country, private insurers and managed care organizations that are regulated by the state must cover diabetes education and nutrition counseling. If you have questions about whether or not your diabetes education will be covered, contact your nearby diabetes education program or dietitian, health care company, your state insurance commissioner's office, the local Medicare office, or the American Diabetes Association.

Restaurant Pitfalls and Strategies for Self-Defense

To eat out healthfully is no small task. You need willpower and perseverance. It's tough enough to eat healthfully in your own house. But even more challenges confront you when you have to pick and choose from a written menu or menu board. You have far less control than when you are in your kitchen. You can't as easily monitor how the food is cooked or see what's added to the food in preparation. However, as you'll learn in the pages ahead, you can put many strategies into action to help you choose healthier restaurant foods.

Healthy restaurant eating is, no doubt, a challenge. In part, that's because there are lots of pitfalls—from mile-high portions to the use of large quantities of fat and salt. The good news is that you can choose to eat healthfully in 99 percent of fast-food restaurants. *Choose* is the critical word here. To choose more carefully, it's important to have a full understanding of the pitfalls of restaurant eating.

Pitfalls of Restaurant Eating

- **You think of restaurant ventures as special occasions.** Yes, once upon a time, people ate in restaurants only to celebrate a birthday, Mother's Day, or an anniversary. That's seldom the case today. Today, restaurant meals for most people are just part of our fast-paced life. They're hardly special occasions. The average American eats four or more meals away from home each week. And personally you may easily top that number. When you eat that many meals away from home each week, your waistline quickly spreads if you treat each meal as a special occasion and/or you finish the portions you are served.

- **You're not the cook.** The person preparing your food is generally out of sight. This means you have less control over how your food is prepared. Your methods of control are to ask questions about the food on the menu, to make special requests to get an item delivered the way you want it, and to practice portion control both when you order and when you eat.

- **Fats are here, there, and everywhere.** Remember, fat makes food taste good and stay moist. Restaurants, therefore, love it. Fat is in high-fat ingredients such as butter, sour cream, or mayonnaise-based sauces; in high-fat foods such as cheese, bacon, or french fries; and in high-fat cooking methods such as deep-fat frying, breading and frying, and sautéing. You need to master the craft of fat detection. You'll get plenty of tips ahead. A bit of good news about fast-food restaurants—the type where you walk up and order—is that you won't be tempted by foods, such as fried Chinese noodles, tortilla chips, or bread and butter, that are brought to you at the table in sit-down restaurants.

- **Sodium can skyrocket.** Along with fat, salt makes food taste good. It is also used in many pre-prepared restaurant foods to keep them safe. Fast-food restaurant foods are notorious for the high sodium content of their foods. Many restaurants pour it aplenty. If you're watching your sodium intake, you'll need to shy away from certain items and make some special requests.

- **Portions are oversized.** Restaurants simply serve too much food. Unfortunately, they and many Americans believe that more is better. The portions are often enough for two. You need to develop and use strategies that help you not overeat. In fast-food restaurants, you can often select from a variety of different serving sizes, such as regular, medium, large, or jumbo. Note that it's often harder to find the small servings and easier to find the large servings. Obviously, they want you to buy more food.
- **Meat (protein) is front and center.** A primary focus of the American diner is summed up in the catch-phrase "Where's the beef?" Whether it is fish, chicken, or beef, the protein often takes center stage in restaurant meals. And most plates contain too much of it. A steak is often 8 oz or more cooked. A chicken breast is often a whole chicken breast. A goal to eat healthier is to put the meat on the side of your plate and fill the rest of your plate with healthier sides—vegetables and whole-grain starches.

Americans Eat Out: How Much and How Often?

An average American today spends almost half of every food dollar on food eaten away from home. In 1950, according to the National Restaurant Association, the average American spent only a quarter of his or her food dollar eating away from home. The average American today eats four or more meals out of the house each week. Lunch is the meal eaten out most often, with dinner a close second. Breakfast is eaten out least often. And men eat out more than women. Fast-food restaurants—from hamburger joints to pizza and sub shops—represent about a quarter of all restaurant meals. As for ethnic food, Americans' favorites are Mexican, Chinese, and Italian.

It is estimated that Americans eat about one-third of their calories away from home. Research shows that more of these calories are from meats, starches, fats, and sugary foods and drinks and that fewer of these calories are from fruits, vegetables, whole grains, and low-fat dairy foods.

Let's face it, restaurant meals—eaten in or out—are just part of dealing with our fast-paced world. You might ask, "Is that a problem if I have diabetes?" The answer is no, as long as you learn to eat healthy restaurant meals most of the time. And remember, whether you eat in the restaurant or take food out to the soccer field, your office, or the kitchen table, you face the same decisions.

In fact, you have to make similar choices in today's supermarkets, because they have begun to look a bit like restaurants, with ready-to-eat parts of meals, complete meals, sandwiches, premade salads, and salad bars. Of course, one advantage in the supermarket is that frequently the nutrition facts stare you in the face. In restaurants, you have to hunt a little more for the nutrition information. Much more information is available from large national fast-food restaurant chains such as the 13 restaurants featured in this book. Less nutrition information is available from national chain sit-down restaurants and even less from independently owned restaurants.

Ten Strategies to Eat Out Healthfully

1. **Develop a can-do attitude.** Too many of us think in negative equations: Eating out equals pigging out; a restaurant meal is a special occasion; eating out means blowing your "diet." These attitudes defeat your efforts to eat healthfully. It's time to develop a can-do attitude about restaurant meals. Build confidence to believe that you can enjoy a healthy meal when you eat out. Slowly begin to change how you order and the types of restaurants in which you choose to eat.

2. **Decide when to eat out—or not.** Take a look at how often you eat out. If your count verges on the excessive, then ask yourself why you eat out so frequently and how you can reduce your restaurant meals. You may find that you eat out more often in fast-food restaurants, especially since they are at your disposal nearly 24/7. Also, if you eat out more frequently, you need to keep splurges to a minimum. If you eat out only once a month, you might take a few more liberties—perhaps with an alcoholic drink or a dessert.

3. **Zero in on the site.** Seek out restaurants that offer at least a smattering of healthier options. Remember, there is an advantage to eating in chain restaurants. You know the menu all too well. This can help you plan ahead, no matter which one of the chain's locations you pop into.

4. **Set your game plan.** On your way to the restaurant—whether it's a quick fast-food lunch or a leisurely weekend dinner—envision a healthy and enjoyable outcome. Plan your strategy, or at least

what you might have if you aren't familiar with the restaurant, before you cross the threshold. Don't become a victim of hasty choices or be swayed by the sights and smells.

5. **Become a well-trained fat detective.** Learn to focus on fats. Fat is the densest form of calories, and it often gets lost in the sauce, so to speak—or on the salad, on the bread, or in the chips. Watch out for high-fat ingredients—butter, mayonnaise-based sauces, or sour cream. Be alert for high-fat foods—cheese, avocado, sausage, and bacon. Steer clear of high-fat preparation methods—frying of any kind. Look out for high-fat dishes—burgers piled high with cheese and bacon, fried chicken sandwiches, salads topped with fried chicken and loaded with salad dressing, or pizza loaded with extra cheese and high-fat meats.

6. **Let your food plan be your guide.** Choose foods with your healthy eating plan in mind. Try to fulfill each food group requirement with menu items, or substitute foods to make your meal complete. For instance, replace a serving of milk or a fruit serving, which are often hard to get in restaurants, with another starch serving so that you will keep your carbohydrate intake consistent—an important diabetes goal.

7. **Practice portion control from the start.** The best way not to eat too much is to order less. Order with your stomach in mind, not your eyes. You need to outsmart the menu to get the right amount of food for you. Take advantage of smaller serving sizes and don't get taken in by meal deals or more food for less money come-ons.

8. **Be creative with the menu.** You outsmart the menu by being creative. You also control portions

by being creative. Remember, no sign at the entrance says, "All who enter must eat a lot of food." Your options are to take advantage of smaller servings and to split menu items if you choose. Consider, for example, splitting a sandwich or salad with your dining partner; eating family- or Asian-style; or mixing and matching two entrées to achieve nutritional balance. For example, in a hamburger chain, split a large burger and split a baked potato filled with broccoli and topped with cheese sauce. In a pizza restaurant, order a medium instead of a large pizza to help you eat fewer slices.

9. **Get foods made to order.** Don't be afraid to ask for what you want, even in a fast-food restaurant. Restaurants today need your business and want you back. Make sure your requests are practical— leave an item such as potato chips off the plate; substitute mustard for mayonnaise on a sandwich; make a sandwich on whole-wheat bread rather than on a croissant; or serve the salad dressing on the side. Restaurants can abide these requests. However, don't expect to have your special requests greeted with a smile at noon in a fast-food restaurant or when you try to remake a menu item. Be reasonable and pleasant.

10. **Know when enough is enough.** Many of us grew up being members of the clean-plate club. Now you need to reserve a membership in the "leave-a-few-bites-on-your-plate club." To keep from overeating, don't order too much, order creatively, and push your plate away when you meet your calorie needs.

Restaurant Dilemmas and Diabetes

Many people who eat restaurant meals have concerns about their health and need to ask questions. So, as a person with diabetes, your questions and special requests are nothing out of the ordinary. However, as someone with diabetes, you deal with dilemmas beyond just the food because of your medication schedule and your blood glucose goals. This section provides you with guidance to face these additional challenges.

Delayed Meals

A big challenge, if you take a diabetes medication that can cause your blood glucose to get too low (see Table 1, p. 20), may be how to manage delayed meals. For example, if you are used to eating lunch between noon and 12:30 pm, how can you safely delay your meal until 1:00 or 1:30 pm when your friends or business associates want to meet? Or what should you do if you want to eat at 7:30 pm on a Saturday night, when your usual dinner time during the week is 6:00 pm?

A big and positive change in the management of diabetes today is that there are new oral blood glucose–lowering medications and new types of insulin that better mesh with the realities of life in the twenty-first century. Several of these medications help your health care providers, diabetes educators, and you work out the best medication schedule to manage

TABLE 1 Diabetes Medications and Hypoglycemia

Diabetes medications that can cause hypoglycemia	Diabetes medications that do not cause hypoglycemia*
Sulfonylureas: Amaryl, Glucotrol, Glucotrol XL, glyburide, glipizide, DiaBeta, Glynase, Micronase	Metformin: Glucophage, Glucophage XR, Riomet
	Alpha-glucosidase inhibitors: Precose and Glyset
Combination pill: Glucovance (combination of metformin and glyburide; the glyburide portion can cause hypoglycemia), Metaglip (combination of metformin and glipizide; the glipizide portion can cause hypoglycemia), Avandaryl (combination of Avandia and Amaryl), and others	Glitazones: Avandia and Actos
	Combination pill: Avandamet (combination of Avandia and metformin), ACTOplus met (combination of Actos and metformin), and others
	Exenatide (Byetta), pramlintide (Symlin)
Meglitinides: repaglinide (Prandin)	
d-phenylalanine: nateglinide (Starlix)	*When any of these medications are used in combination with ones that can cause hypoglycemia, hypoglycemia can occur.
Insulin: all types, injected or inhaled (Exubera)	

your blood glucose while allowing you the flexibility you need to live your life in the manner that best suits your needs. What's important in developing a medication plan is that you communicate your lifestyle and schedule to your health care providers and diabetes educators. If they don't know your habits, then they are less able to help you develop a medication plan that suits you.

The biggest concern in delaying meals is whether you have taken a diabetes medication that can cause your blood glucose to go too low if you don't eat on time. Prior to the availability of new blood glucose–lowering oral medications and newer insulins, this was more of a concern than it is today. But it is certainly still a concern for you if your blood glucose can get too low. On page 20 is a list of the diabetes medications that can cause blood glucose to go too low (cause hypoglycemia) and those that cannot. If you take one or more of the medications that can cause low blood glucose, then you need to pay special attention to your meal times.

Keep in mind that several of the newer diabetes medications that can cause hypoglycemia are rapid-acting, such as the insulins lispro (Humalog), aspart (Novolog), and glulisine (Apidra), as well as inhaled insulin (Exubera) and the oral pills Prandin and Starlix. Their job is to quickly lower your blood glucose after you eat. If you take one of these medications along with other medications that are not likely to cause low blood glucose, take these rapid-acting medications a few minutes before you start to eat rather than at your usual meal time. (See the section on rapid-acting insulins, below.)

If you take a pre-mixed combination of insulin, such as 70/30 or 75/25, or just take insulin twice a day, such as a dose of NPH or Lente and regular or rapid-acting insulin, it becomes more important for you to eat on time to prevent low blood glucose. A disadvantage of these insulin regimens is that they are not as easy to adjust when you eat meals at a different time than usual. If you regularly need more flexibility in your schedule, then talk to your health care providers and diabetes educators about your needs. Today, there are much more flexible insulin regimens, including the use of an insulin pump or the use of the longer-acting insulins glargine (Lantus) or detemir (Levemir) with one of the rapid-acting insulins (Humalog, Novolog, or Apidra) or the use of inhaled insulin (Exubera). Most of the injectable insulins are available for use in pens.

Practical Tips for Using Rapid-Acting Insulin with Restaurant Meals

More and more people who take insulin are on a flexible insulin regimen. Usually, they take Lantus once or twice a day and rapid-acting or inhaled insulin just before they eat. More people are also using insulin pumps. These so-called flexible insulin regimens can make insulin dosing for restaurant meals easier.

Recent observations suggest that rapid-acting insulin doesn't get absorbed and lower blood glucose as quickly as practitioners first believed when it came on the market in 1996. Today, most experts agree that the maximum blood glucose–lowering effect of rapid-acting insulin occurs closer to one and a half to two hours after an injection rather than in 45 minutes. If this is true for you, and you've tested this out by doing some after-meal blood glucose checks, the optimal time to take rapid-acting insulin is about 10 to 15 minutes before you eat, rather than with the first bite or 15 minutes after you start to eat. This is especially true if your blood glucose is higher than your target before your meal.

Another big key to blood glucose management is to give yourself enough insulin to cover the rise of blood glucose from the food you eat. Like many people, you may find yourself in a reactive mode when it comes to dosing insulin. This means that you take it in response to high blood glucose rather than taking enough insulin just before a meal to cover the rise of blood glucose in the hours after you eat. Blood glucose usually rises to its high point one to two hours after a meal that contains a moderate amount of fat and protein. Your blood glucose should be back down to your pre-meal target four to five hours after you eat. It may take longer if you eat large meals or you eat foods and meals that are high in fat and meat. Experts agree that it's much harder for you to bring a high blood glucose back down into the normal range than to control the rise of blood glucose by taking sufficient insulin before eating or at least when you know the amount of carbohydrate you will eat.

Although taking rapid-acting insulin 10 to 15 minutes before a meal and carefully calculating your dose according to the carbohydrate you will eat are ideal for blood glucose management, you may not always be able to do so, for one reason or another, when you eat restaurant meals. These practical tips can help you keep your blood glucose on target when you eat restaurant meals.

High blood glucose (>180 mg/dl) before a meal: Take some rapid-acting insulin a half hour before your meal to give the insulin time to lower your blood glucose. It might take longer than this to come down, but at least you will have given the insulin a running start at lowering your blood glucose before it goes up again when you eat.

Low blood glucose before a meal: If your blood glucose is low before a meal (below about 70 mg/dl), wait to take your insulin or treat the low blood glucose. If you choose to wait to give the insulin, give the carbohydrate about 15 minutes to raise your blood glucose before you take the insulin to cover your food. Don't wait any longer, because the action curve will be delayed.

Uncertain carbohydrate intake: If you don't know how much carbohydrate you will eat at a meal, consider splitting your rapid-acting insulin dose. Take enough insulin 10 to 15 minutes before the meal to cover a minimum amount of carbohydrate that you know you will eat, say 30 to 45 grams. Then, as the meal goes on and you know how much more carbohydrate you will eat, take more insulin to cover that amount. This method is easiest if you are on an insulin pump or if you use an insulin pen.

Drawn-out meals: Pump users who plan to have a long, drawn-out restaurant meal and/or a meal that is higher in fat may want to consider using one of the optional bolus delivery tools on their insulin pump. Most insulin pumps allow you to deliver a bolus over time (extended or square wave) rather than all at once or to deliver some insulin immediately and some over the next few hours (combination or dual wave).

Learn from your experiences: Because of the large variation in responses to blood glucose from food and insulin among individuals, you can learn how to fine-tune your blood glucose management by recording your experiences for future reference. Keep notes of your responses to various foods and activities in a notebook, computer file, or your logbook. Chart this information: foods you eat and the amounts, the amount of insulin you take to cover the food, your blood glucose levels before and after you eat (2 hours, 4 hours, 6 hours), and any lessons you learn to apply the next time around. Although blood glucose management can be difficult, your personal database can help you adjust to the many different situations you encounter in everyday life.

Steps to Take If Low Blood Sugar Is Possible

If you will delay a meal and you take a longer-acting pill or insulin that can cause your blood glucose to get too low, take precautions to prevent this. Follow these steps.

Check your blood glucose at the usual time of your meal.

- If it is high (>150 mg/dl*), you can wait a short time before you eat without concern. But do check again if you feel your blood glucose is getting too low before your meal.
- If your blood glucose level is around your pre-meal goal (90–130 mg/dl) and you feel it will fall too low before you get to eat, eat some carbohydrate (start with 10 to 15 grams) to make sure your blood glucose doesn't go too low before your meal.
- If you delay your meal more than one hour and your blood glucose is around your pre-meal goal, you may need to eat more than 10 to 15 grams of carbohydrate to keep it from going too low before your meal.

It is always a smart idea to keep easy to carry and eat carbohydrate foods in places such as your desk, briefcase, purse, locker, or glove compartment. Also, it is good to carry glucose tablets. They help you treat an impending low blood glucose before it gets too low and are the most desirable and effective form of treatment for low blood glucose. After all, you never know what will happen in restaurants. As the saying goes, "It's better to be safe than sorry."

---

*The numbers used for blood glucose values in this book are based on plasma glucose goals, not whole blood. Today, most blood glucose meters read results as plasma, not whole blood.

Suggested foods that are easy to carry and contain carbohydrate are dried fruit, cans of juice, pretzels, milk, yogurt, gum drops, gummy bears, or snack crackers. Check the nutrition facts label on the food to determine the amount equivalent to 15 grams of carbohydrate.

If your blood glucose is lower than 70 mg/dl and/or you feel the symptoms of low blood glucose, then you should use 15 grams of some source of carbohydrate to treat your hypoglycemia. Try to eat your meal soon after.

These suggestions offer you general rules of thumb. Check with your health care providers or diabetes educator to learn the best alternatives for you based on your diabetes medication plan. But if your diabetes medication plan is not fitting with your lifestyle, recognize that there are alternatives.

Alcohol

Clearly there are numerous reasons not to drink alcohol. Alcohol is high in calories (unhealthy calories). It can cause low blood glucose if you take an oral diabetes medication or insulin that can cause low blood glucose. It can lead to health problems with overuse, can slow your responses, and can be dangerous if you drink and drive. However, if you are meeting your blood glucose and blood lipid goals and you drink sensibly, there is no reason you cannot enjoy some alcohol. And a common time to drink alcohol is when you eat in a restaurant. Here's how to drink smartly with diabetes.

Tips to Sip By

- Don't drink when your blood glucose is below 70 mg/dl or you have symptoms of hypoglycemia.

- Remember that alcohol can cause low blood glucose after you drink it (if your medicine is working hardest and/or you need to eat). It can continue to cause low blood glucose 8–12 hours after you drink it, especially if you drink in excess, take too much medicine, or don't eat enough.
- Don't drink on an empty stomach. Either munch on a carbohydrate source (popcorn or pretzels) as you drink or wait to drink until you get your meal.
- Alcohol can also make blood glucose too high. High blood glucose can be caused by the calories from carbohydrate in the alcoholic beverage, such as wine or beer, or in a mixer, such as orange juice.
- Avoid mixers that add lots of carbohydrates and calories—tonic water, regular soda, syrups, juices, and liqueurs.
- Check your blood glucose level to help you decide whether you should drink and when you need to eat something.
- Wear or carry identification that states you have diabetes.
- Sip a drink to make it last.
- At a meal, have a noncaloric, nonalcoholic beverage by your side to quench your thirst. Try water, club soda, or diet soda.
- If you do not take a diabetes medicine that can cause low blood glucose and you have some pounds to shed, you can substitute an alcoholic drink for fats in your meal plan.
- If you do not have to lose weight, then just have an occasional drink and don't worry about the extra calories.
- Do not drive for several hours after you drink alcohol. Never drink and drive.

Sugars and Sweets

It is common to want a sweet dessert to end some restaurant meals. As you know by now, you can fit sweets into your diabetes food plan as long as you substitute them for other foods or compensate for their extra carbohydrates, fat, and calories with your diabetes medicines to keep your blood glucose close to normal. To set healthy goals with sweets, you also need to consider your weight and blood fats. Work with a dietitian to figure out how to fit sweets into your meal plan. In the meantime, here are a few pointers.

Hints for Sweet Tooths

- Prioritize your personal diabetes goals. Which is most important for you: managing your blood glucose, losing weight, or lowering your blood fats? Your priorities dictate how you strike a balance with sugars and sweets.
- Choose a few favorite desserts. Decide how often to eat them and how to fit them into your meal plan.
- Perhaps it is best for you to limit desserts just to when you eat in restaurants. That way you keep sweets out of your home.
- Split a dessert in a restaurant or take half home if possible. Portions are generally too big.
- Take advantage of smaller portions available in restaurants or ice cream spots—*kiddie*, *small*, and *regular* are the words to look for.
- Use the nutrition information you find in this book and information you find in restaurants to learn about the calorie, carbohydrate, fat, saturated fat, and cholesterol content of desserts.

- When you eat a sweet, check your blood glucose about two hours later to see how it has been affected. Then check again at four or five hours to see if your blood glucose is back down to your pre-meal target. You might find, for instance, that because of the fat content, the same quantity of ice cream raises your blood glucose more slowly than does frozen yogurt, which contains less fat and more carbohydrate.
- Keep an eye on your A1C (your longer-range blood glucose measure) and your blood fat (lipid) levels to see whether eating more sweets leads to a worsening in these numbers.

These are basic guidelines and suggestions to deal with diabetes restaurant dilemmas. Each person with diabetes is different. Talk with your health care provider and diabetes educator to get information pertinent to the way you manage your diabetes.

Restaurants Help or Hinder Your Healthy Eating Efforts

The pendulum has swung back and forth over the last few decades regarding whether restaurants support or harm your efforts to eat healthily. Here's what has evolved. During the 1980s and early 1990s, when the voices of people concerned about what they ate and about their health were loud, restaurants developed healthier options. Lower-calorie and lower-fat menu items were introduced. Restaurateurs willingly made lower-fat milk and reduced-calorie salad dressings available. Some restaurants even marked their menus with little hearts or other notations to indicate which menu items met specific health criteria.

The pendulum then swung back in the late 1990s and early 2000s. McDonald's dropped the McLean hamburger, and the first generation of entrée salads went by the wayside. Taco Bell's Border Lights line bombed in the late 1990s because it was introduced after the bubble burst on healthier restaurant alternatives. We were back in the era of giant burgers, supersized meals, and more all-you-can-eat buffets.

In the last few years, some restaurant chains have again begun offering healthy alternatives, in part because of interest in low-carb diets and as a way of responding to the chants from health experts about the childhood and adult obesity and type 2 diabetes epidemics. For example, McDonald's has stopped offering to supersize portions. Entrée salads are standard fare at most burger chains, and it's easier to find a few fruit offerings here and there. Perhaps the restaurant that has played up its healthier options the most is Subway.

Unfortunately, a majority of Americans still cast all health and nutrition cares to the wind when they set foot in any restaurant—even a fast-food restaurant they frequent a couple times a week. You can see where that is leading us. Today, over 65 percent of American adults are overweight and 41 million Americans have pre-diabetes, which puts them at risk for type 2 diabetes. About 21 million Americans have diabetes, and 90 to 95 percent of them have type 2 diabetes.

The "no cares" nutrition attitude makes it harder for people who are health conscious. But don't feel pessimistic. Lower-fat milk, reduced-calorie salad dressings, and lower-fat frozen desserts are still widely available, and there's a greater ease in making special requests. With skills and a bit of fortitude, you can eat healthfully at most restaurants. Granted, you still have to pick and choose among the menu offerings.

Remember, too, that your voice still matters. You can make a difference.

Chains That Give the Nutrition Lowdown

The amount of nutrition information available for restaurant foods has exploded with the popularity of the Internet. It is now relatively easy to access nutrition information for the fast-food hamburger chains —from the large McDonald's and Burger King to the smaller Carl's Jr. and Sonic. Among the categories of restaurants and chains that make nutrition information available on their Web sites are those selling pizza, chicken, Mexican food, desserts and ice cream, subs and sandwiches, and donuts and bagels. This book provides the nutrition information for the largest 13 fast-food chain restaurants. If this book piques your curiosity, supplement it with the *Guide to Healthy Restaurant Eating* (also by Hope Warshaw and published by the ADA), which gives nutrition information for the top 60 restaurant chains across America.

The types of restaurants that, for the most part, either do not have or do not provide nutrition information are chain sit-down restaurants. Several of these restaurants are all too happy to give you nutrition information about their few healthier items. But somehow they don't have the information or are unwilling to disclose the nutrition information for the complete menu.

Why don't some restaurants provide nutrition information? There are a few reasons. First, it's expensive to obtain nutritional analyses on all menu items. Second, restaurants that do not provide information tend to change their menus frequently. As soon as they printed nutrition information, it would need to be revised. Third, they want you to stay blindfolded to the nutrition lowdown on their foods. An important point here is that you—a person with diabetes concerned about your health—need to keep asking for nutrition information at restaurants that don't give it.

How to Get the Latest Nutrition Lowdown

If you do not find a particular restaurant chain in this book or there is a new menu item introduced for a restaurant that is included, here are a few hints on how to get the nutrition information.

- If you have access to the Internet, use it. Usually the nutrition information is tucked into the menu information.
- If you don't have Internet access, ask for nutrition information at the store location you frequent. You might get lucky and have a nutrition pamphlet put right into your hands. Sometimes they have run out or just don't keep them in stock. Make sure you check the date on the nutrition pamphlet to be sure it is current.
- If the restaurant does not have the information, ask where you can call or write for it. You might need to call or write the corporate headquarters and have them send you a pamphlet.
- If you have a question about the nutrition content or ingredients used in a few items, contact the company either through the Internet or by phone.

A Bit of Help from the Government

The nutrition facts panel on most canned and packaged foods in the supermarket hardly seems new. But they have only been in their current format for just over a decade. The Nutrition Labeling and Education Act (NLEA), which is the federal legislation that changed the nutrition label and increased the number of foods with information, requires restaurants to comply with several aspects of this law. Restaurants must provide nutrition information to customers when nutrition and health claims are made on signs and placards.

If any restaurant makes a health claim about a food—that it is "low-fat," for instance—the nutrition information has to comply with the meaning of the term according to the NLEA. This helps you know that when you see the word "healthy" to describe a can of beans or a fast-food sandwich, it has the same meaning. Restaurants from small one-unit sandwich shops to McDonald's have to abide by these regulations. Table 2 (see page 36) gives terms you might see on restaurant menu items and their definitions.

The law permits restaurants to make

- specific claims about a menu item's nutritional content.
- one of the approved health claims about the relationship between a nutrient or food and a disease or health condition. The criteria to make the health claim must be met.

If the restaurant makes a nutrition or health claim, it must provide you with the nutrition information to back it up. The claim can be substantiated by a nutrition database, nutrition information in the cookbook from which the recipe was made, or another source that provides nutrition information. Further, restaurants do not have to give you the information in the nutrition label format you are familiar with from the supermarket. They can provide it in any format they choose.

Now there is a move afoot to require chain restaurants with more than a certain number of outlets to provide nutrition information. Legislation has been introduced in several states and at the federal level in both the House and the Senate. The Center for Science in the Public Interest has done a good job of promoting the need for this information. More information about this topic is available at www.cspinet.org.

TABLE 2 Meaning of Nutrition Claims* on Restaurant Menus, Signs, and Placards

Nutrition Claim	Meaning
Cholesterol-Free	Less than 2 mg of cholesterol per serving and 2 g or less of saturated fat per serving
Low-Cholesterol	20 mg or less of cholesterol per serving and 2 g or less of saturated fat per serving
Fat-Free	Less than 0.5 g of fat per serving
Low-Fat	3 g or less of fat per serving
Light or Lite	Cannot be used by restaurants as a nutrient content claim, but can be used to describe a menu item, such as "lighter fare" or "light size"
Sodium-Free	Less than 5 mg of sodium per serving
Low-Sodium	140 mg or less of sodium per serving
Sugar-Free	Less than 0.5 g of sugar per serving
Low-Sugar	May not be used as a nutrient claim
Healthy	The food item is low in fat, low in saturated fat, has limited amounts of cholesterol and sodium, and provides significant amounts of one or more key nutrients—vitamins A and C, iron, calcium, protein, or fiber.
Heart Healthy (These claims will indicate that a diet low in saturated fat and cholesterol may reduce the risk of heart disease.)	The item is low in fat, saturated fat, and cholesterol, and provides without fortification (added nutrients) significant amounts of one or more key nutrients—vitamins A and C, iron, calcium, protein, or fiber. OR The item is low in fat, saturated fat, and cholesterol, and provides without fortification (added nutrients) significant amounts of one or more key nutrients—vitamins A and C, iron, calcium, protein—and is a significant source of soluble fiber.

*The definitions of these claims are the same as those used for food labels in the supermarket.

Tips to Eat Healthier: Breakfast, Burgers, Pizza, and More

Healthy Tips for Breakfast and Snack Restaurants

- Choose coffee without cream, whole milk, or sugar. They add fat and empty calories. Use lower-fat or fat-free milk and sweeten with a sugar substitute. Today you often have three choices—Splenda, Equal, and Sweet 'N Low.
- Try half of a soft-baked pretzel as an accompaniment to a salad or as a snack.
- Opt for one of the light bagel spreads, but keep in mind that they are hardly calorie- or fat-free. Spread them thinly.
- Cake donuts have slightly less fat than yeast donuts.
- Consider half of a bagel, muffin, scone, or sweet bread. For many people, that's enough carbohydrate and calories. If a whole-grain variety is available, grab it.
- Do eat breakfast. Skipping breakfast just keeps your engine in low gear and may help you rationalize overeating at meals during the rest of the day. Plus, if you take diabetes medications that can cause low blood glucose, skipping breakfast is not a smart move.
- In breakfast sandwiches, choose ham or cheese and pass on bacon or sausage. Have these fillings on a

bagel or an English muffin rather than on a high-fat biscuit or croissant.

- Read the fine print when you see the words low-fat, fat-free, and sugar-free. They don't mean that there are no calories or no carbohydrate. In fact, some of these foods can contain more carbohydrate and/or more calories than the regular food.
- If jam or jelly is an option, take it. Jams and jellies have no fat. Spread them thinly all the same.
- The fancy coffees and teas—both hot and iced, from mochas to frappuccinos to chais—are not just coffee and tea. The whole milk, half-and-half, and whipped cream add calories and fat. The sugar from syrups adds calories and carbohydrate with no nutrition. These drinks can contain upwards of 300 calories for even the small size. You've got better ways to spend your calories.

Get It Your Way

- Order bagel spreads on the side so that you can control how much is spread.
- Order butter or margarine on the side.
- Opt for fat-free milk in specialty coffees.
- Order a sandwich on a bagel or roll, not on a high-fat croissant.

Healthy Tips for Burger Chains

- Zero in on the words *regular*, *junior*, *small*, or *single*. These mean small portions.
- Try lower-calorie ketchup, mustard, or barbecue sauce as an option to higher-fat mayonnaise or special sauce.

- Limit the high-fat toppers and add-ons—cheese, bacon, and special sauce.
- Look for healthier items—entrée and side salads, baked potatoes, healthy soups, cut fruit, and 100% juice.
- Walk in rather than drive through. If you eat and drive, you hardly realize food has passed your lips.
- Order less food to start. Remember, you can go back and get more in a flash.
- Want fries? Go ahead, but split a small or medium order.

Get It Your Way

- Avoid the busy times. This way you'll get your food your way with a smile on the order taker's face.
- Be ready to wait. Fast-food restaurants are not set up for special requests.
- Ask for simple changes: leave off the special sauce or mayonnaise; hold the pickles, bacon, or cheese; or hold the salt on the french fries.

Healthy Tips for Chicken Chains

- You are better off going skinless. If the chicken is served with skin, take the skin off and save some fat grams. You'll also lighten up on cholesterol and saturated fat.
- If there's enough for two meals, ask for a take-out container and split the meal into two before you dig in.
- To keep fat grams and calories down, go with the quarter white meat. Wings and thighs have the most fat.
- Order à la carte to pick and choose between the healthier items—a piece of white meat chicken,

corn, beans, etc.—and skip the biscuit, hushpup-pies, and other high-fat side items.

- If you are going to eat the meal at home, a better buy (price- and healthwise) is a whole chicken and several sides. That way you—rather than the server—can decide on your portions.
- Split a quarter of a chicken meal and add an extra side or two. This keeps the protein portion where it should be, at about 2–3 ounces.

Get It Your Way

- Ask to have the skin removed if you can't trust yourself to do it.
- Ask the server to take the wing off the breast.
- Ask for the gravy, butter, or salad dressing on the side.

Healthy Tips for Pizza Chains

- If you need to count calories carefully, stick with the thin crust and load up on the veggies.
- If your favorite chain does not publish nutrition information, check the nutrition information for similar items from two other pizza chains. These will give you ballpark figures to base your choice on.
- If your dining partner wants not-so-healthy pizza toppings, order healthier toppings on one half and let your partner handle the other.
- If you count grams of carbohydrate, make sure the slices you eat are average. If they are bigger or smaller, change your carbohydrate estimate and insulin dose (if you take insulin) based on your best guess for the size of the slices you eat.

- Order just enough for everyone at the table, to avoid that just-one-more-piece syndrome.
- If you know a few extra pieces will be left over, package them up before you take your first bite.
- Try an appetizer side portion of pasta, split an order with your dining partner, or stash a portion in a take-home container before you lift your fork to your mouth.
- Along with pizza or pasta, crunch on a healthy garden salad to fill you up and not out.
- The red pepper flakes you'll probably find sitting right on your table add zip to your pizza, pasta, or salad without adding calories.

Healthy Pizza Toppings

part-skim cheese	sliced tomatoes
chicken	green peppers
spinach	ham
onions	broccoli
Canadian bacon	mushrooms
pineapple	

Not-So-Healthy Pizza Toppings

extra cheese	pepperoni
anchovies	several types of cheese
sausage	bacon

Get It Your Way

- Ask your pizza maker to go light on the cheese and heavy on the veggies.
- Request a half-order of pasta if you don't have someone to split it with.
- Remember to order your salad dressing on the side.

Healthy Tips for Sandwich and Sub Shops

- Opt for the smaller size sandwiches when possible—6" sub, small or regular size sandwich.
- To keep your sodium meter on low, go light on or hold the pickles and olives.
- To keep the fat level down, skip the oil and mayonnaise. Opt for vinegar and mustards. You get lots of flavor with next to no fat.
- Choose to have your sandwich made on whole-grain bread if it's available.
- Complement a sub or sandwich with a healthier side than a fried snack food (potato chips, tortilla chips, and the like). For some crunch, try a side salad, popcorn, baked chips, or pretzels.
- Ask to have large subs cut into two. Pack up half for another day.
- In sandwich shops, order a cup of broth-based vegetable or bean soup or a side garden salad. They'll fill you up and not out.
- A Greek salad and a piece of pita bread make a moderate-carbohydrate and light-on-protein meal. Ask for dressing on the side.
- Pack a piece of fruit from home to bring to the sub or sandwich shop.

Get It Your Way

- Hold the mayonnaise and oil. Substitute mustard or vinegar.
- Ask the sub maker to go light on the meat and heavy on the lettuce, onions, tomatoes, and peppers.
- Hold the cheese.
- Ask for the salad dressing on the side.

Healthy Tips for Mexican Restaurants

- If the fried tortilla chips greet you when you sit down, hands off. Send them back or at least to the opposite side of the table. But hold on to the salsa!
- Order à la carte to have less food in front of you and to pick and choose among the healthier offerings.
- Use extra salsa and other hot sauces to add flavor with very few calories.
- Use salsa or another hot sauce as a salad dressing.
- Don't feel that you must order an entrée. Choose an appetizer or side dish to control your portions.
- Take advantage of ordering à la carte. Mix and match a healthy meal.
- As a starter, try a cup of black bean soup or chili to fill you up and not out.
- Make a bowl of black bean soup or chili the main course with a salad on the side.
- Look for menu items that use soft tortillas rather than crispy fried ones. For example, choose a burrito or an enchilada rather than a taco or a chimichanga.
- Fajitas are great to split. There's always enough for two.
- Split a side dish—Mexican rice, refried beans, or black beans—to get more carbohydrates and fiber.
- Take advantage of light or nonfat sour cream if it's served.

Get It Your Way

- Hold the guacamole, cheese, and sour cream, or ask for them on the side.
- If a menu item is served with melted cheese, request a light helping.

- Substitute black beans for refried beans (if available).
- Ask for extra tomatoes and lettuce.
- Request extra salsa or other zesty, low-calorie toppers.

Healthy Tips for Ice Cream Shops

- Choose among the healthier toppings— fresh fruit, granola, nuts, or raisins.
- Take advantage of the variety of portions—from kiddie to multiple scoops.
- Don't think kiddie size is just for kids. It's a great small size for calorie and carbohydrate counters too.
- Order one dessert and two spoons. Just a few bites will often quiet your sweet tooth.

Get It Your Way

- Choose low-fat or fat-free frozen yogurt, light ice cream, or sorbet and order kiddie or small portions. Options are aplenty for healthful eating.

Put Your Best Guess Forward

When you've got the nutrition facts in hand, it makes knowing the nutrients you eat a snap. And the listings in this book help a great deal when you choose to eat in one of the 13 fast-food chains whose information is provided in the pages ahead. The ADA also publishes a larger book, *Guide to Healthy Restaurant Eating*, with nutrition information for more than 60 national chains.

The reality is, however, that nutrition facts are simply not available from some of the restaurants in which you may choose to eat. They might be sit-down chain restaurants unwilling to provide information, smaller local chains, or independent single-location restaurants that are unlikely to have any nutrition information. Assessing the nutrient content of what you eat in these restaurants is more of a challenge. The following tips will help you learn to put your best guess forward.

Tips to Put Your Best Guess Forward

- Have measuring equipment at home and use it. Have a set of measuring spoons and measuring cups, as well as an inexpensive food scale. Weigh and measure foods at home sometimes. Do this regularly as you familiarize yourself with the portions you should eat. Then on occasion, say once a month, weigh and measure foods, especially the starches, fruits, and meats. Weighing and measuring foods at home regularly helps you keep portions in control and helps you more precisely estimate them in restaurants. Estimating with the precise portion size helps you estimate the nutrient content most correctly.

■ Use these "handy" hand guides to estimate portions:
- Tip of the thumb (to first knuckle)—1 teaspoon
- Whole thumb—1 tablespoon
- Palm of your hand—3 ounces (this is the portion size of cooked meat that most people need at a meal). Other 3-ounce portion guides: the size of a deck of regular size playing cards or the size of a household bar of soap.
- Tight fist—1/2 cup
- Loose fist or open handful—1 cup
  Note: These guidelines hold true for most women's hands, but some men's hands are much larger. Check the size of your hands out for yourself with real weighing and measuring equipment.

■ Use the scales in the produce aisle of the supermarket to educate yourself about the servings of food you may be served in a restaurant, such as baked white or sweet potatoes, an ear of corn, or a banana. Weigh individual pieces of these foods. Check out how many ounces in a typical potato or an ear of corn like the ones you may be served in a restaurant. Note that you are weighing these foods raw, but their weight doesn't change that much when cooked.

■ If there are no data for a particular restaurant you frequent, use the information available from other similar restaurants in this book or in the *Guide to Healthy Restaurant Eating* (published by the ADA). If you want to get a feel for the nutrient content of a food like french fries, baked potato, stuffing, pizza, or bagels, look at the serving size and nutrition information for those foods in restaurants that are included. You might want to take a few examples and then do an average. For example, if you regularly eat at a local pizza shop rather than a national chain and they have no nutrition information, take the nutrition information from this book for two slices of medium-sized, regular-crust cheese pizza from three restaurants. Then do an average. You will come pretty close to the nutrition content of the two slices of cheese pizza you eat.

- You can also use the nutrition information from the nutrition facts of foods in the supermarket to estimate what you might eat in a restaurant. You might find some similar foods in the frozen or packaged convenience foods area. Again, take a couple of examples and then average.

- If you regularly eat particular ethnic foods for which you find no nutrition information, you might want to get a few cookbooks out of the library (or use your own) that contain recipes for the foods you enjoy. Then use a nutrient database or a book with nutrition information (see pages 49–50) to determine the estimated nutrient content for each ingredient. Do this for a couple of similar recipes. Then get an average to help you estimate the nutrient content of what you are eating in the restaurant. This might work well for ethnic foods such as Indian, Mexican, or Chinese.

Most people regularly eat just 50 to 100 foods, including restaurant foods. People tend to frequent the same restaurants and order similar items. For this reason, it makes sense to spend some time estimating the nutrient content of your favorite restaurant foods for which nutrition information is not available. Once you have this figured out, put it in a notebook or develop a computer file that you print out and keep with you.

Keep in mind that most restaurants serve portions that are larger than most average-sized people need to eat. So, even if you choose healthy foods that combine to make a healthy meal, you will likely also need to limit the amount you eat. Portion control is clearly not an easy task. Learn some techniques by reading the "Ten Strategies to Eat Out Healthfully" on pages 15–17.

A word to the wise: Avoid all-you-can-eat restaurants and other settings that simply promote overeating, such as hotel breakfast buffets or salad or food bars. This is best if you don't have much willpower or it bothers you to think that the restaurant is making money on you because you will not walk out feeling like a stuffed turkey. However, if you feel these settings work well because they help you control portions, use them to your advantage.

If you frequently eat particular items in large chain restaurants for which nutrition information is not available in this book, contact the restaurants. Although several restaurants were unwilling to provide the nutrition information for all their items for this book, they noted that if a customer contacted them, they would provide information for several items.

Resources for Nutrition Information of Foods

Books

The Diabetes Carbohydrate and Fat Gram Guide, by Lea Ann Holzmeister, RD, CDE. American Diabetes Association, 3rd edition, 2005, 603 pages. This book provides the carbohydrate count, as well as other nutrition information, for thousands of foods, including fruits, vegetables, and other produce; meats, poultry, and seafood; desserts; many foods you know by their brand name; frozen entrées; and more.

The Doctor's Pocket Calorie, Fat, and Carb Counter, by Allan Borushek. Allan Borushek and Associates (a new book is published each year). This book lists calorie, fat, and carbohydrate information for thousands of basic and brand-name foods. (See www.calorieking.com to order the book or to download food and restaurant databases.)

Calories and Carbohydrates, by Barbara Kraus. Signet, 15th edition, 2003, 496 pages. Carbohydrate and calorie counts for more than 8,500 items are included in this food dictionary. It covers brand-name and basic foods of every variety.

The Corinne T. Netzer Carbohydrate Counter, by Corinne T. Netzer. Dell, 7th edition, 2001, 496 pages. This book features carbohydrate counts for thousands of foods, including fresh and frozen produce, dairy products, breads, grains, pastas, sweets, fast foods, and more.

Internet

www.ars.usda.gov/ba/bhnrc/ndl. From this Web site, the United States National Agricultural Library, you can search or download a nutrient database of 6,000 basic foods for free.

www.calorieking.com
www.nutritiondata.com
www.dietfacts.com

How This Book Works for You

Close but Not Exact

You should be aware that the nutrition information from restaurants is close but not exact. Many restaurants state that their nutrition information is based on the specified ingredients and preparation. However, the same restaurant has locations all over the country, and different regions purchase their ingredients and foods from different food wholesalers. For example, a Wendy's in California might purchase lettuce, tomatoes, and hamburger buns from one food supplier, whereas a Wendy's in Connecticut will buy foods from another company. The nutrition analysis of these items is close, but not identical. However, it is close enough to help you to make food decisions and manage your blood glucose.

Restaurant foods are also prepared by different people. Even in the same restaurant, on different days you might get more or less cheese on your pizza, more pickles or ketchup on your hamburger, or fewer pieces of chicken on your entrée salad. Wherever humans are involved, portions aren't exact. Consider these differences if one day you notice that your blood glucose goes up more or less than you expect from a restaurant meal you've eaten again and again.

Beverages and Condiments

There are two categories of items that are not listed separately in the information provided for each restaurant. The first is beverages. Regularly sweetened drinks, such as carbonated beverages (soda or pop), lemonade, noncarbonated fruit drinks, and the like, are not listed individually because, from a nutrition standpoint, they are loaded with sugar and provide almost no nutritional value. Most restaurants also serve a similar variety of noncaloric beverages as well as milk and orange juice. To avoid repeating information on the same products, we've put the nutrition information for the most commonly served regular and diet beverages in Table 3 on pages 54 and 55.

The second category of items not listed for individual restaurants is common condiments, such as ketchup, mustard, mayonnaise, and honey. Don't despair; we've put the nutrition information for these condiments in Table 4 on pages 56–58.

The Nutrition Numbers Ahead

All the nutrition information from the 13 largest fast-food chains is in the pages ahead. Whether you use the diabetes exchange system, carbohydrate or calorie counting, or some other meal planning system that works for you, the numbers are here. Here is the nutrition information you'll find, in this order:

- Calories
- Fat (in grams) and
  - Percentage of calories from fat. Look at this in relation to grams of fat. Keep in mind that the

percentage of calories from fat might be high, but the grams of fat might be low, or vice versa.

- Saturated fat (in grams). Saturated fat is a type of fat that raises blood cholesterol levels. Try to keep your saturated fat intake to 10 percent or less of your total calories.
- Trans fat (in grams). Trans fat is an unhealthy type of fat. Some restaurants provide this information.
- Cholesterol (in milligrams)
- Sodium (in milligrams)
- Carbohydrate (in grams)
  - Dietary fiber (in grams). Dietary fiber is a component of carbohydrate. Generally, Americans don't eat enough dietary fiber. Try to eat 20–35 grams of dietary fiber each day.
- Protein (in grams)
- Food servings/exchanges. Servings and exchanges are virtually the same. They have been calculated using the 2003 *Exchange Lists for Meal Planning*, published by the ADA and the American Dietetic Association, and *Diabetes Meal Planning Made Easy*, 3rd edition, published by the ADA in 2006.

A "best-fit" approach was used to calculate servings or exchanges. There is no one right way to fit restaurant foods into your meal plan. Figuring out which food group the grams of carbohydrate come from is the biggest challenge to figuring servings or exchanges. Here's how it works in this book: When the grams of carbohydrate come from a starch—potatoes, bread, or starchy vegetables, for example—the servings or exchanges are called starches. If the carbohydrate comes from vegetable, fruit, or milk, the servings or exchanges are designated as such.

TABLE 3 Nutrition Information for Beverages

Beverage	Amount	Cal.	Fat (g)	Sat. Fat (g)	Chol. (mg)	Sod. (mg)	Carb. (g)	Pro. (g)	Servings/Exchanges
Beer (regular)	12 oz	140	0	0	0	11	13	1	n/a*
Beer (light)	12 oz	99	0	0	0	18	5	1	n/a*
Coffee, black (regular and decaffeinated)	8 oz	5	0	0	0	4	1	0	free
Coke (regular)	12 oz	144	0	0	0	6	43	0	3 carb
Coke (diet)	12 oz	1	0	0	0	6	0	0	free
Iced Tea (unsweetened)	12 oz	4	0	0	0	6	1	0	free
Liquor (any type)	1 1/2 oz	96	0	0	0	0	0	0	n/a*
Lemonade (regular)	12 oz	160	0	0	0	0	42	0	3 carb
Milk (whole)	8 oz	150	8	5	33	120	12	8	1 whole milk
√Milk (reduced-fat/2%)	8 oz	120	5	3	18	122	12	8	1 low-fat milk

Milk (low-fat/1%)	8 oz	102	2	2	12	107	12	8	1 fat-free milk, 1/2 fat
✓Milk (fat-free)	8 oz	83	0	0	4	126	12	8	1 fat-free milk
Milk, chocolate (low-fat)	8 oz	157	3	2	8	152	26	8	1 fat-free milk, 1 carb
✓Apple juice	8 oz	117	0	0	0	7	29	0	2 fruit
✓Orange juice	8 oz	110	0	0	0	2	25	2	2 fruit
Pepsi (regular)	12 oz	144	0	0	0	6	43	0	3 carb
Pepsi (diet)	12 oz	1	0	0	0	6	0	0	free
Sprite (regular)	12 oz	148	0	0	0	3	37	0	2 1/2 carb
Sprite (diet)	12 oz	1	0	0	0	6	0	0	free
Tea (hot, nothing added)	8 oz	2	0	0	0	7	1	0	free
Wine, white	6 oz	120	0	0	0	9	1	0	n/a*
Wine, red	6 oz	120	0	0	0	114	3	1	n/a*

*n/a= not available. Talk to your diabetes educator or health care provider about whether you can work alcoholic beverages into your meal plan and how to do so.
✓=Healthiest Bets

TABLE 4 Nutrition Information for Condiments

Condiment	Amount	Cal.	Fat (g)	Sat. Fat (g)	Chol. (mg)	Sod. (mg)	Carb. (g)	Pro. (g)	Servings/Exchanges
Bacon, thinly sliced	1 slice	36	3	1	5	101	0	2	1 fat
Butter	1 t	30	4	2	10	39	0	0	1 fat
Cheese, American	1-oz slice	106	9	6	27	405	1	6	1 high-fat meat
Cheese, Swiss	1-oz slice	107	8	5	26	74	1	8	1 high-fat meat
Cheese, mozzarella, whole-milk	1/4 cup shredded/1 oz	80	6	4	22	106	1	6	1 medium-fat meat
Cream Cheese (regular)	1 T	50	5	3	15	45	1	1	1 fat
Cream Cheese (light)	1 T	30	3	2	5	80	1	2	1/2 fat
Half & Half	1/2 oz/1 T	20	2	1	6	6	1	0	free
Honey	1 t	22	0	0	0	0	6	0	1/2 carb
Honey Mustard	1 t	15	1	n/a	n/a	75	2	0	free

Ketchup	1 T	16	0	0	0	137	4	0	free
Margarine (regular stick)	1 t	34	4	1	0	44	0	0	1 fat
Margarine (regular tub)	1 t	34	4	1	0	51	0	0	1 fat
Margarine (light)	1 t	17	2	0	0	17	0	0	free
Mayonnaise (regular)	1 T	100	11	2	8	78	0	0	2 fat
Mayonnaise (light)	1 T	40	4	0	5	15	1	0	1 fat
Mustard	1 t	5	0	0	0	65	0	0	free
Non-Dairy Creamer	1/2 oz/1 T	16	1	0	0	5	2	0	free
Olive Oil	1 t	40	5	2	0	0	0	0	1 fat
Pancake Syrup (regular)	1 T	50	0	0	0	13	13	0	1 carb
Pancake Syrup (light)	1 T	25	0	0	0	56	7	0	1/2 carb
Pancake Syrup (low-calorie)	1 T	23	0	0	0	57	6	0	1/2 carb

(Continued)

TABLE 4 **Nutrition Information for Condiments** (*Continued*)

Condiment	Amount	Cal.	Fat (g)	Sat. Fat (g)	Chol. (mg)	Sod. (mg)	Carb. (g)	Pro. (g)	Servings/Exchanges
Relish, pickle-type	1 T	19	0	0	0	164	5	0	free
Salsa, tomato-based	1 T	3	0	0	0	112	1	0	free
Sour Cream (regular)	1 T	26	3	2	5	6	1	0	1/2 fat
Sour Cream (light)	1 T	18	1	0	5	10	1	1	free
Soy Sauce	1 t	3	0	0	0	343	1	0	free
Vinegar (all types)	1 t	2	0	0	0	0	1	0	free

n/a=not available

One food group in the 2003 *Exchange Lists for Meal Planning* is called the "other carbohydrate" group. This group contains foods such as sweets, frozen desserts, spaghetti sauce, jam, and maple syrup, to name a few. The calories and carbohydrates in many of these foods come from simple sugars. Therefore, in calculating the servings or exchanges for this book, we've called foods that fit into the "other carbohydrate" group "carb." Exchanges for fast-food shakes and frozen and regular desserts, for example, are calculated as carbs.

When it comes to meat dishes, the servings or exchanges were calculated based on the group that the meat itself fits into, regardless of how it's prepared. For example, fish fillet sandwiches and chicken fingers are considered to fall into the lean meat group even though they have a lot of fat by the time they are served. On the other hand, sausage in any form is classified as a high-fat meat because that's the food group sausage fits into.

It is worth noting that some restaurants that provide nutrition information also provide exchanges. These were not used in this book. We calculated exchanges and servings based on ADA methodology. We have often found inconsistencies between the restaurant's exchange calculations and the ones obtained using ADA guidelines.

Putting It All Together

Perhaps one of the hardest parts of meal planning is figuring out how to put together healthy, well-balanced meals. This is a particular challenge in fast-food restaurants. To show you how to design healthier restaurant meals, we've put together two sample meals for these 13 restaurants (except for Baskin Robbins). Please note that the criteria might be less strict than what you would consider for a healthy meal at home. That's because restaurant meals tend to be higher in calories and fat. Sometimes, even though the meal shown is a combination of the restaurant's healthiest offerings, it was nearly impossible to meet the criteria below, especially for fat and sodium. Do keep in mind that you can make special requests to have higher-fat or -sodium ingredients left out, so that the items that you eat are healthier. We applied the following criteria to put together the meals.

The Light & Lean Choice

- 400–700 calories (based on about 1,200–1,600 calories per day)
- 30–40 percent of calories from fat
- Trans fat as close to none as possible
- 100–200 milligrams of cholesterol (total per day should be 300 milligrams or less)
- 1,000–1,800 milligrams of sodium (total per day should be no more than 2,300 milligrams)

The Healthy & Hearty Choice

- 600–1,000 calories (based on about 1,800–2,400 calories per day)
- 30–40 percent of calories from fat
- Trans fat as close to none as possible
- 100–200 milligrams of cholesterol (total per day should be 300 milligrams or less)
- 1,000–1,800 milligrams of sodium (total per day should be no more than 2,300 milligrams)

Healthiest Bets

With nutrition information in hand, we've also made it easy for you to zero in on healthier restaurant offerings. We've marked these "Healthiest Bets" with a check mark (✔). Remember, foods that are not marked as Healthiest Bets are not necessarily foods you should never eat. Healthiest Bets just steer you toward healthier choices.

When you're putting together healthy meals, don't look at only the Healthiest Bets. Mix and match healthier and less healthy foods to make up overall healthy meals. Also keep in mind that if you split or share some less healthy bets, such as shakes, desserts, or fried items, they then fit into Healthiest Bets. That's why you'll see some Healthiest Bets and some less healthy items mixed and matched in the sample meals for each restaurant. What's most important is that you eat a healthy balance over the course of the day and from week to week. So if you want a juicy hamburger and french fries for lunch one day a month, go ahead and enjoy.

The Healthiest Bets were chosen on the basis of the following criteria developed by the author:

■ Breakfast entrées (including sandwiches): Less than 400 calories per serving, with less than 15 grams of fat (3 fat exchanges [about 30 percent fat]) and 1,000 milligrams of sodium.

■ Lunch or dinner entrées, including entrée salads: Less than 600–750 calories, with less than 20 grams of fat (4 fat exchanges [about 30 percent fat]) and 1,000 milligrams of sodium.

■ Pizza, sandwiches, hamburgers, etc.: Less than 500 calories per reasonable serving (for example, 2 slices of pizza), 20 grams of fat (4 fat exchanges [about 30 percent fat]), and 1,000 milligrams of sodium.

- Side items: For items such as fruit, vegetables (raw and cooked), grains, legumes, starches, and meats, no more than 5 grams of fat (1 fat exchange). For fried items, such as french fries, hash browns, chicken pieces, fried chicken, onion rings, and potato chips, less than 10 grams of fat (2 fat exchanges); less than 500 milligrams of sodium per serving.

- Soups: Less than 10 grams of fat (2 fat exchanges) and 1,000 milligrams of sodium per serving.

- Salad dressings, cream cheeses, spreads, and condiments: Less than 50 calories, 5 grams of fat (1 fat exchange), and 250 milligrams of sodium per tablespoon.

- Breads (such as rolls, biscuits, bagels, bread, croissants, donuts, muffins, pretzels, and scones): Less than 400 calories, 10 grams of fat (2 fat exchanges), and 800 milligrams of sodium per serving.

- Desserts: Less than 300 calories, 10 grams of fat (2 fat exchanges), and 30 grams of carbohydrate per serving.

- Beverages (such as milk, juice, milk shakes, and special coffees): Less than 300 calories, 30 grams of carbohydrate, 5 grams of fat (1 fat exchange), and 400 milligrams of sodium. (Coffee and diet beverages, though minimal in calories, were not checked as Healthiest Bets.)

Bon Appetit!

Section 2:
Fast-Food Restaurants

Arby's

www.arbys.com

Light & Lean Choice

1 Jr. Roast Beef Sandwich
Curly Fries (1/2 small order)

Calories	442	Cholesterol (mg) 29
Fat (g)	20	Sodium (mg) 1,135
% calories from fat	...41	Carbohydrate (g) 54
Saturated fat (g)	 6	Fiber (g) 4
Trans fat (g)	.... 1.5	Protein (g) 18

Exchanges: 3 1/2 starch, 2 medium-fat meat, 1 fat

Healthy & Hearty Choice

1 Santa Fe Salad with Grilled Chicken
Light Buttermilk Ranch Dressing (3 T)
1 Blueberry Muffin

Calories	709	Cholesterol (mg) 98
Fat (g)	27	Sodium (mg) 1,165
% calories from fat	...34	Carbohydrate (g) 80
Saturated fat (g)	 9	Fiber (g) 7
Trans fat (g)	 0	Protein (g) 35

Exchanges: 4 starch, 2 vegetables, 3 lean meat, 3 fat

(*Continued*)

Arby's

	Amount	Cal.	Fat (g)	% Cal. Fat	Sat. Fat (g)	Trans Fat (g)	Chol. (mg)	Sod. (mg)	Carb. (g)	Fiber (g)	Pro. (g)	Servings/Exchanges
BREAKFAST												
French Toastix	1	312	13	37	2	0	0	192	44	1	6	3 starch, 2 fat
Sausage Patty	1	210	20	85	7	0	40	480	0	0	6	1 high-fat meat, 2 fat
Syrup	1	78	0	0	0	0	0	25	20	0	0	1 1/2 carb
BREAKFAST BISCUIT												
Bacon	1	340	21	55	6	0	13	1028	29	1	9	2 starch, 1 high-fat meat, 1 1/2 fat
Bacon, Egg & Cheese	1	461	28	54	8	0	169	1446	30	1	17	2 starch, 2 high-fat meat, 2 fat
Chicken	1	417	23	49	5	1	17	1240	39	1	15	2 starch, 1 medium-fat meat, 3 fat

	Amount	Cal.	Fat (g)	% Cal. Fat	Sat. Fat (g)	Trans Fat (g)	Chol. (mg)	Sod. (mg)	Carb. (g)	Fiber (g)	Prot. (g)	Exchanges/Choices
Ham	1	316	17	48	4	0	13	1240	29	1	13	2 starch, 1 medium-fat meat, 1 fat
Ham, Egg & Cheese	1	437	23	47	6	0	169	1658	31	1	20	2 starch, 2 high-fat meat, 2 fat
Plain	1	273	15	49	4	0	1	786	28	1	5	2 starch, 2 fat
Sausage	1	436	27	55	9	0	32	1160	28	1	10	2 starch, 1 high-fat meat, 3 fat
Sausage Gravy	1	961	68	63	14	0	12	3755	107	1	19	7 starch, 1 high-fat meat, 10 fat
Sausage, Egg & Cheese	1	557	38	61	11	0	187	1579	30	1	18	2 starch, 2 high-fat meat, 3 fat
BREAKFAST CROISSANT												
Bacon & Egg	1	337	22	58	10	0	187	651	23	1	11	1 1/2 starch, 1 high-fat meat, 2 fat

(Continued)

✔ = Healthiest Bets

BREAKFAST CROISSANT *(Continued)*	Amount	Cal.	Fat (g)	% Cal. Fat	Sat. Fat (g)	Trans Fat (g)	Chol. (mg)	Sod. (mg)	Carb. (g)	Fiber (g)	Pro. (g)	Servings/Exchanges
Bacon, Egg & Cheese	1	378	22	52	10	0	198	850	23	1	14	1 1/2 starch, 2 high-fat meat, 1 fat
✔Ham & Cheese	1	274	12	39	7	0	53	842	22	1	13	1 1/2 starch, 1 medium-fat meat, 1 fat
Ham, Egg & Cheese	1	434	24	49	10	0	343	1282	25	1	22	1 1/2 starch, 2 high-fat meat, 3 fat
✔Plain	1	190	10	47	6	0	30	190	21	1	3	1 1/2 starch, 2 fat
Sausage 'n Egg	1	433	32	66	13	0	206	784	23	1	12	1 1/2 starch, 1 high-fat meat, 4 fat
Sausage, Egg & Cheese	1	475	32	60	13	0	216	982	23	1	15	1 1/2 starch, 2 high-fat meat, 4 fat
BREAKFAST SOURDOUGH												
Bacon, Egg & Cheese	1	437	16	32	5	0	174	1220	40	2	20	3 starch, 2 high-fat meat

Item	Amount	Cal.	Fat (g)	% Fat Cal.	Sat. Fat (g)		Chol. (mg)	Sod. (mg)	Carb. (g)			Exchanges
Egg & Cheese	1	392	12	27	3	0	166	1058	40	2	17	2 1/2 starch, 1 medium-fat meat, 1 1/2 fat
Ham, Egg & Cheese	1	679	35	46	11	0	354	2104	42	6	34	3 starch, 3 medium-fat meat, 3 fat
Sausage, Egg & Cheese	1	514	27	47	8	0	186	1232	40	2	19	3 starch, 2 medium-fat meat, 2 fat

BREAKFAST WRAP

Item	Amount	Cal.	Fat (g)	% Fat Cal.	Sat. Fat (g)		Chol. (mg)	Sod. (mg)	Carb. (g)			Exchanges
Bacon, Egg & Cheese	1	515	29	50	8	2	165	1367	50	2	16	3 starch, 2 high-fat meat, 2 1/2 fat
Ham, Egg & Cheese	1	568	31	49	10	2	183	1929	51	2	24	3 1/2 starch, 2 high-fat meat, 2 1/2 fat
Sausage, Egg & Cheese	1	689	45	58	15	2	202	1849	50	2	21	3 1/2 starch, 2 high-fat meat, 4 fat

(Continued)

✔ = Healthiest Bets

	Amount	Cal.	Fat (g)	% Cal. Fat	Sat. Fat (g)	Trans Fat (g)	Chol. (mg)	Sod. (mg)	Carb. (g)	Fiber (g)	Pro. (g)	Servings/Exchanges
CHICKEN NATURALS												
Chicken Tenders	5 pc	723	35	43	6	3	80	2268	54	4	48	3 1/2 starch, 5 lean meat, 4 fat
Chicken Tenders	3 pc	434	21	43	4	2	48	1361	32	2	29	2 starch, 3 lean meat, 2 fat
CHICKEN NATURALS SANDWICHES												
Chicken Bacon & Swiss - Crispy	1	624	29	41	7	1	68	1320	52	2	36	3 1/2 starch, 4 lean meat, 3 fat
Chicken Bacon & Swiss - Grilled	1	462	17	33	4	0	25	1333	38	2	38	2 1/2 starch, 4 lean meat, 1 fat
Chicken Cordon Bleu - Crispy	1	650	31	42	6	1	74	1548	49	2	40	3 1/2 starch, 4 medium-fat meat, 2 fat

	Amount	Cal.	Fat (g)	% Cal. Fat	Sat. Fat (g)	Trans Fat (g)	Chol. (mg)	Sodium (mg)	Carb. (g)	Fiber (g)	Pro. (g)	Servings/Exchanges
Chicken Cordon Bleu - Grilled	1	488	19	35	4	0	32	1561	35	2	42	3 starch, 4 medium-fat meat
Chicken Fillet - Crispy	1	576	30	46	5	1	52	901	50	3	30	3 1/2 starch, 3 lean meat, 3 1/2 fat
✔ Chicken Fillet - Grilled	1	414	17	36	3	0	9	913	36	3	32	2 starch, 3 lean meat, 1 1/2 fat
SW Chipotle Chicken - Crispy	1	680	37	48	10	1	77	1228	51	3	38	3 1/2 starch, 4 lean meat, 4 fat
SW Chipotle Chicken - Grilled	1	517	25	43	8	0	34	1241	37	3	39	2 1/2 starch, 4 lean meat, 2 fat
DESSERTS												
✔ Gourmet Chocolate Cookie	1	200	10	45	4	2	15	213	26	0	2	1 1/2 carb, 2 fat
DESSERTS - TURNOVERS												
Apple w/ icing	1	380	12	28	3.5	6	0	200	64	2	4	4 carb, 1 fruit
Apple w/out icing	1	250	10	36	3	6	0	200	35	2	4	1 carb, 1 fruit, 2 fat

✔ = Healthiest Bets

(Continued)

DESSERTS - TURNOVERS *(Continued)*	Amount	Cal.	Fat (g)	% Cal. Fat	Sat. Fat (g)	Trans Fat (g)	Chol. (mg)	Sod. (mg)	Carb. (g)	Fiber (g)	Pro. (g)	Servings/Exchanges
Cherry w/ icing	1	380	12	28	3.5	6	0	200	64	2	4	3 carb, 1 fruit, 2 fat
Cherry w/out icing	1	250	10	36	3	6	0	200	35	2	4	1 carb, 1 fruit, 2 fat
MARKET FRESH SALADS												
Chicken Club	1	504	26	46	8	2	209	1235	32	5	33	1 1/2 starch, 2 veg, 4 medium-fat meat, 1 1/2 fat
✔Martha's Vineyard w/out dressing	1	277	8	25	4	0	72	454	24	5	26	1/2 starch, 3 veg, 3 very-lean meat, 1/2 fat
Santa Fe w/ Crispy Chicken w/out dressing	1	499	23	41	8	2	59	1231	42	7	30	1 1/2 starch, 3 veg, 3 medium-fat meat, 1 fat
✔Santa Fe w/ Grilled Chicken w/out dressing	1	305	11	32	6	0	78	621	21	6	30	1/2 starch, 3 veg, 3 lean meat, 1 fat

MARKET FRESH SANDWICHES

Corned Beef Reuben	1	606	33	49	9	1	83	1849	55	3	34	3 1/2 starch, 5 medium-fat meat, 1 fat
Roast Beef and Swiss	1	777	41	47	13	2	89	1743	73	5	37	5 starch, 3 high-fat meat, 2 fat
Roast Ham and Swiss	1	705	31	39	8	1	63	2103	75	5	36	5 starch, 3 high-fat meat, 1/2 fat
Roast Turkey and Swiss	1	725	30	37	8	1	91	1788	75	5	45	5 starch, 4 medium-fat meat, 1/2 fat
Roast Turkey Reuben	1	611	30	44	8	1	94	1429	56	3	44	3 1/2 starch, 5 medium-fat meat, 1 fat
Ultimate BLT	1	779	45	51	11	1	51	1571	75	6	23	3 starch, 2 high-fat meat, 5 fat

MARKET FRESH WRAP

Chicken Salad with Pecans	1	638	38	53	10	0	74	1199	48	8	30	3 starch, 3 medium-fat meat, 4 fat

(Continued)

✔ = Healthiest Bets

MARKET FRESH WRAP *(Continued)*	Amount	Cal.	Fat (g)	% Cal. Fat	Sat. Fat (g)	Trans Fat (g)	Chol. (mg)	Sod. (mg)	Carb. (g)	Fiber (g)	Pro. (g)	Servings/Exchanges
Roast Turkey Ranch & Bacon	1	700	37	47	11	1	109	2215	44	4	49	3 starch, 6 medium-fat meat, 1 fat
Southwest Chicken	1	567	29	46	9	1	88	1451	42	4	36	3 starch, 4 medium-fat meat, 1/2 fat
Ultimate BLT	1	648	44	61	11	1	51	1530	45	5	23	3 starch, 2 high-fat meat, 5 fat
MUFFINS												
Blueberry	1	320	12	33	2	0	20	490	49	1	4	3 starch, 2 fat
OTHER SANDWICHES												
✔ Arby's Melt	1	302	12	35	4	1	30	921	36	2	16	2 starch, 1 high-fat meat, 1 fat
Bacon, Beef 'n Cheddar	1	521	27	46	9	2	64	1573	45	2	27	3 starch, 2 high-fat meat, 2 fat

	Amount										Exchanges/Choices
Beef 'n Cheddar	1	445	21	42	6	1	51	1274	44	2	22	3 starch, 2 medium-fat meat, 2 fat
Fish Sandwich	1	569	36	56	7	0	60	995	63	3	22	4 starch, 2 medium-fat meat, 4 fat
French Dip	1	391	16	36	6	1	28	1282	37	3	26	2 1/2 starch, 2 medium-fat meat, 1 fat
French Dip and Swiss	1	473	18	34	7	1	79	1679	38	3	32	2 1/2 starch, 4 medium-fat meat
Ham and Swiss Melt	1	275	6	19	2	0	27	1118	35	1	18	2 starch, 2 lean meat
Hot Ham and Cheese	1	304	7	20	2	0	35	1420	35	1	23	2 starch, 2 lean meat
✔ Jr. Ham and Swiss Melt	1	211	5	21	1	0	23	873	23	1	14	1 1/2 starch, 1 medium-fat meat
Sourdough Roast Beef Melt	1	355	14	35	5	1	30	1047	40	2	18	3 starch, 1 high-fat meat, 2 fat

(Continued)

✔ = Healthiest Bets

OTHER SANDWICHES *(Continued)*	Amount	Cal.	Fat (g)	% Cal. Fat	Sat. Fat (g)	Trans Fat (g)	Chol. (mg)	Sod. (mg)	Carb. (g)	Fiber (g)	Pro. (g)	Servings/Exchanges
Sourdough Roast Ham Melt	1	380	13	30	3	0	31	1280	39	2	19	2 1/2 starch, 1 high-fat meat, 2 fat
ROAST BEEF SANDWICHES												
✔ Jr. Roast Beef	1	272	10	33	4	0	29	740	34	2	16	2 starch, 1 lean meat, 1 1/2 fat
Large Roast Beef	1	547	28	46	12	2	102	1869	41	3	42	3 starch, 4 medium-fat meat, 1 1/2 fat
Medium Roast Beef	1	415	21	45	9	1	73	1379	34	2	31	2 starch, 4 medium-fat meat
✔ Regular Roast Beef	1	320	14	39	5	1	44	953	34	2	21	2 1/2 starch, 3 medium-fat meat
Super Roast Beef	1	398	19	42	6	1	44	1060	40	2	21	3 starch, 2 medium-fat meat, 1 1/2 fat

✔ Swiss Melt	1	303	12	35	4	1	29	919	37	2	16	3 1/2 starch, 1 high-fat meat, 1 fat

SAUCES AND CONDIMENTS

✔ Arby's Sauce Packet	1	15	0	0	0	0	0	180	4	0	0	free
✔ BBQ Dipping Sauce	2 T	40	0	0	0	0	0	350	10	0	0	1/2 carb
Bronco Berry Sauce	4 T	120	0	0	0	0	0	35	30	0	0	2 carb
Buttermilk Ranch Dressing	4 T	290	30	93	5	1	25	580	3	0	1	6 fat
Cheddar Cheese Sauce (for Fries)	3 T	60	5	75	1	1.5	0	360	4	0	1	1 fat
✔ Horsey Sauce Packet	1 T	62	5	72	1	0	5	173	3	0	0	1 fat
✔ Light Buttermilk Ranch Dressing	4 T	112	6	48	1	0	0	472	13	0	1	1 starch, 1 fat
✔ Marinara Sauce	5 T	30	1.5	45	0	0	0	160	4	0	0	1/2 starch
✔ Raspberry Vinaigrette	2.5 oz	194	14	64	2	0	0	387	18	0	0	1 carb, 2 1/2 fat

✔ = Healthiest Bets

(Continued)

SAUCES AND CONDIMENTS *(Continued)*	Amount	Cal.	Fat (g)	% Cal. Fat	Sat. Fat (g)	Trans Fat (g)	Chol. (mg)	Sod. (mg)	Carb. (g)	Fiber (g)	Pro. (g)	Servings/Exchanges
Santa Fe Ranch Dressing	3 T	296	31	94	5	0	21	692	4	0	1	6 fat
Seasoned Tortilla Strips	1 T	71	3	38	0.5	0	0	25	9	0	1	1/2 carb, 1/2 fat
✔Sliced Almonds	1 T	81	7	77	0	0	0	0	2	1	4	1 1/2 fat
Tangy Southwest Sauce	4 T	330	35	95	5	0	30	370	5	0	1	1/2 carb, 7 fat
✔Three Pepper Sauce Packet	1	22	1	40	0	0	0	140	3	0	0	free
S H A K E S												
Chocolate - Large	1	660	17	23	10	0	45	450	110	0	17	7 carb, 3 1/2 fat
Chocolate - Regular	1	510	13	22	8	0	35	360	83	0	13	5 1/2 carb, 2 1/2 fat
Jamocha - Large	1	650	17	23	10	0	45	510	107	0	17	7 carb, 3 1/2 fat
Jamocha - Regular	1	500	13	23	8	0	35	390	81	0	13	5 carb, 2 1/2 fat
Strawberry - Large	1	650	17	23	10	0	45	460	107	0	16	7 carb, 3 1/2 fat
Strawberry - Regular	1	500	13	23	8	0	35	360	81	0	13	5 carb, 2 1/2 fat

Vanilla - Large	1	650	17	23	10	0	45	470	107	0	16	7 carb, 3 1/2 fat
Vanilla - Regular	1	500	13	23	8	0	35	370	82	0	13	5 1/2 carb, 2 1/2 fat

SIDES

Broccoli & Cheese Baked Potato	1	535	22	37	11	2	48	784	73	8	12	5 starch, 4 fat
✔Butter & Sour Cream Baked Potato	1	495	24	43	15	0	56	167	65	6	8	4 starch, 5 fat
Curly Fries - large	1	631	37	52	7	6	0	1476	73	7	8	5 starch, 5 fat
Curly Fries - medium	1	406	24	53	4	4	0	949	47	5	5	3 starch, 4 fat
Curly Fries - small	1	338	20	53	4	3	0	791	39	4	4	2 1/2 starch, 3 fat
✔Deluxe Baked Potato	1	645	32	44	19	1	91	346	67	6	20	4.5 starch, 1 high-fat meat, 4 fat
Home-style Fries - large	1	566	37	58	7	5	0	1029	82	6	6	5 1/2 starch, 5 fat
Home-style Fries - medium	1	377	25	59	4	4	0	686	55	4	4	4 starch, 3 fat

✔ = Healthiest Bets

(Continued)

SIDES *(Continued)*	Amount	Cal.	Fat (g)	% Cal. Fat	Sat. Fat (g)	Trans Fat (g)	Chol. (mg)	Sod. (mg)	Carb. (g)	Fiber (g)	Pro. (g)	Servings/Exchanges
Home-style Fries - small	1	302	20	59	4	3	0	549	44	3	3	3 starch, 1 1/2 fat
Jalapeno Bites	5	305	21	61	9	2	28	526	29	2	5	2 starch, 4 fat
Large Onion Petals	1	828	57	61	9	2	2	831	88	5	10	6 starch, 8 fat
Loaded Potato Bites	5	353	22	56	7	1	13	800	27	2	11	3 starch, 4 fat
Mozzarella Sticks	4	426	28	59	13	2	45	1370	38	2	18	3 1/2 starch, 1 high-fat meat, 4 fat
Potato Cakes	3	369	28	68	5	5	0	587	39	3	3	2 1/2 starch, 5 fat
Regular Onion Petals	1	331	23	62	4	1	1	332	35	2	4	3 starch, 4 fat
Sour Cream Baked Potato	1	393	12	27	7	0	25	50	65	6	8	4 starch, 2 fat
SUBS												
Italian	1	622	33	47	7	1	51	1986	48	3	24	3 starch, 2 high-fat meat, 3 fat

Philly Beef and Swiss	1	670	35	47	11	1	90	1942	46	4	36	3 starch, 3 lean meat, 5 fat
Roast Beef	1	723	42	52	11	2	89	2210	46	3	35	3 starch, 3 lean meat, 6 fat
Turkey	1	633	30	42	3	1	75	2029	47	3	35	3 starch, 3 lean meat, 4 fat

T.J. CINNAMON'S

Chocolate Twist	1	250	12	43	4	0	5	110	31	2	4	2 starch, 2 1/2 fat
Cinnamon Roll	1	507	10	17	4	0	7	373	73	4	10	5 starch, 2 fat
Cinnamon Twist	1	260	14	48	5	4	5	190	33	1	3	2 starch, 3 fat
Pecan Sticky Bun	1	688	22	28	5	0	7	420	91	5	12	6 starch, 4 fat
T.J. Icing	1	117	5	38	2	1	8	50	18	0	1	1 carb
T.J. Mocha Chill	1	306	7	20	4	0	29	214	48	1	11	3 carb

✔ = Healthiest Bets

Baskin Robbins

www.baskinrobbins.com

No meals are provided for this chapter because these foods are usually eaten as a snack or in addition to a meal.

(*Continued*)

Baskin-Robbins

BREEZE

	Amount	Cal.	Fat (g)	% Cal. Fat	Sat. Fat (g)	Trans Fat (g)	Chol. (mg)	Sod. (mg)	Carb. (g)	Fiber (g)	Pro. (g)	Servings/Exchanges
Kiwi Banana Creamy Bold	16 oz	480	1	1	0	0	0	95	119	4	5	6 carb, 2 fruit
Kiwi Banana Creamy Bold	24 oz	710	1.5	1	0	0	5	150	176	7	8	8 carb, 4 fruit
Kiwi Bold	16 oz	340	0	0	0	0	0	30	87	3	1	4 1/2 carb, 1 fruit
Kiwi Bold	24 oz	470	0.5	1	0	0	0	40	120	4	1	6 carb, 2 fruit
Kiwi Creamy Bold	24 oz	620	1	1	0	0	5	150	152	4	7	8 carb, 2 fruit
Kiwi Creamy Bold	16 oz	440	0.5	1	0	0	0	95	107	3	4	6 carb, 1 fruit
Mango Banana Creamy Bold	16 oz	480	1.5	2	0	0	0	75	116	5	3	6 1/2 carb, 1 fruit
Mango Banana Creamy Bold	24 oz	720	2.5	3	0	0	5	120	172	5	8	9 1/2 carb, 2 fruit

Mango Bold	16 oz	340	1	2	0	0	0	10	84	2	1	4 1/2 carb, 1 fruit
Mango Bold	27 oz	470	1.5	2	0	0	0	15	116	2	1	6 1/2 carb, 1 fruit
Strawberry Banana Creamy Bold	16 oz	490	1.5	2	0	0	0	75	121	5	5	7 carb, 1 fruit
Strawberry Banana Creamy Bold	24 oz	730	1.5	1	0		5	120	178	7	9	10 carb, 2 fruit
Strawberry Citrus	16 oz	350	1	2	0	0	0	10	89	3	1	5 carb, 1 fruit
Strawberry Citrus	24 oz	480	1	1	0	0	0	15	122	4	2	6 carb, 2 fruit
Strawberry Citrus Creamy Bold	16 oz	450	1	2	0	0	0	75	109	3	5	6 carb, 1 fruit
Strawberry Citrus Creamy Bold	24 oz	630	1.5	2	0		5	120	154	4	8	8 carb, 2 fruit
Wild Mango Creamy Bold	16 oz	440	1.5	3	0	0	0	75	104	2	4	6 carb, 1 fruit
Wild Mango Creamy Bold	24 oz	640	2	2	0		5	120	148	3	7	8 carb, 2 fruit

(*Continued*)

✔ = Healthiest Bets

CAPPUCCINO BLASTS

	Amount	Cal.	Fat (g)	% Cal. Fat	Sat. Fat (g)	Trans Fat (g)	Chol. (mg)	Sod. (mg)	Carb. (g)	Fiber (g)	Pro. (g)	Servings/Exchanges
Cappuccino Blast Decaf or Regular w/ whipped cream	16 oz	320	14	39	9	0	55	110	44	0	6	2 starch, 1 carb, 3 fat
Cappuccino Blast Decaf or Regular w/ whipped cream	24 oz	480	21	39	13	0	80	160	67	0	9	2 1/2 starch, 2 carb, 3 1/2 fat
Cappuccino Blast Low Fat Decaf or Regular w/ whipped cream	16 oz	220	2	8	1.5	0	10	115	45	0	6	2 starch, 1 carb
Cappuccino Nonfat Blast	16 oz	210	0	0	0	0	5	120	45	0	7	2 starch, 1 carb
Chocolate w/ whipped cream	24 oz	680	19	25	12	0.5	65	210	123	0	10	5 starch, 3 carb, 2 fat
Chocolate w/ whipped cream	16 oz	450	12	24	8	0	45	140	81	0	6	3 starch, 2 carb, 1 1/2 fat

	Amount	Cal	Fat (g)	% Cal. Fat	Sat. Fat (g)	Trans Fat (g)	Chol. (mg)	Sodium (mg)	Carb. (g)	Fiber (g)	Pro. (g)	Exchanges/Choices
Decaf or regular	24 oz	460	19	37	12	0	75	150	66	0	9	2 starch, 2 carb, 3 1/2 fat
Decaf or regular	16 oz	300	12	36	7	0	45	95	43	0	6	2 starch, 1 carb, 1 1/2 fat
Mintopia	24 oz	530	22	37	14	1	70	180	78	1	10	3 starch, 2 carb, 4 fat
Mintopia	16 oz	360	16	40	10	0.5	45	125	52	1	7	2 1/2 starch, 1 carb, 2 1/2 fat
Mocha Blast	24 oz	540	18	30	12	0	70	140	87	0	8	3 1/2 starch, 2 carb, 3 fat
Mocha Blast	16 oz	350	12	30	7	0	45	90	57	0	5	2 1/2 starch, 1 carb, 2 fat
Mocha Blast w/ whipped cream	16 oz	370	13	31	8	0	50	100	58	0	6	2 1/2 starch, 1 carb, 2 fat
Mocha Blast w/ whipped cream	24 oz	560	20	32	13	0	80	150	88	0	8	4 starch, 2 carb, 3 fat
Turtle Blast	24 oz	710	23	29	13	0.5	70	500	121	0	10	5 starch, 3 carb, 3 1/2 fat
FROZEN YOGURT												
✔Chocolate Nonfat Soft Serve	1/2 cup	120	0	0	0	0	0	85	25	1	4	1 1/2 carb

✔ = Healthiest Bets

(Continued)

FROZEN YOGURT *(Continued)*	Amount	Cal.	Fat (g)	% Cal. Fat	Sat. Fat (g)	Trans Fat (g)	Chol. (mg)	Sod. (mg)	Carb. (g)	Fiber (g)	Pro. (g)	Servings/Exchanges
Maui Brownie Low Fat	1/2 cup	210	4	17	1.5	0	10	140	41	2	6	2 1/2 carb, 1 fat
✔Peppermint Nonfat Soft Serve	1/2 cup	110	0	0	0	0	0	75	24	0	4	1 1/2 carb
Perils of Praline Low Fat	1/2 cup	190	3.5	16	1.5	0	5	170	37	1	5	2 1/2 carb, 1/2 fat
Raspberry Cheese Louise Low Fat	1/2 cup	190	4	18	2.5	0	10	150	36	1	5	2 carb, 1 fat
✔Raspberry Nonfat Soft Serve	1/2 cup	110	0	0	0	0	0	75	25	0	4	1 1/2 carb
Vanilla Nonfat	1/2 cup	150	0	0	0	0	5	105	32	0	6	2 carb
✔Vanilla Nonfat Soft Serve	1/2 cup	110	0	0	0	0	0	80	23	0	4	1 1/2 carb
ICE CREAM CAKE												
Chocolate Chip/Devil's Food	2/3 cup	330	18	49	8	0	55	240	40	1	5	3 carb, 3 fat

Chocolate Ice Cream/ Chocolate Roll	1/2 cup	290	15	46	6	0	40	340	41	2	4	3 carb, 2 1/2 fat
Chocolate Ice Cream/ Devil's Food	3/4 cup	410	23	5	11	0	70	320	51	2	6	3 1/2 carb, 4 fat
Mint Chocolate Chip/ Devil's Food	1/2 cup	290	18	55	8	0	50	200	33	1	4	2 carb, 3 fat
Mint Chocolate Ice Cream/ Chocolate Roll	1/2 cup	290	14	43	6	0	45	240	36	2	5	2 carb, 3 fat
Oreo Cookies 'n Cream Ice Cream	2/3 cup	300	16	48	9	1	50	180	35	1	5	2 carb, 3 fat
Oreo Cookies 'n Cream/ Devil's Food	3/4 cup	430	23	48	10	0.5	65	390	55	1	7	3 1/2 carb, 4 fat
Oreo's 'n Cream/ White Cake	1/2 cup	300	14	42	7	0	45	270	40	1	5	3 carb, 2 fat

✔ = Healthiest Bets

(Continued)

ICE CREAM CAKE (Continued)	Amount	Cal.	Fat (g)	% Cal. Fat	Sat. Fat (g)	Trans Fat (g)	Chol. (mg)	Sod. (mg)	Carb. (g)	Fiber (g)	Pro. (g)	Servings/Exchanges
Pralines 'n Cream/ Devil's Food	3/4 cup	430	20	41	8	0	50	380	65	1	6	4 carb, 3 fat
Pralines 'n Cream/ White Sponge Cake	1/2 cup	300	16	48	6	0	40	280	49	1	5	3 carb, 2 1/2 fat
Vanilla Ice Cream	1/2 cup	290	18	55	11	0	70	80	39	0	5	2 1/2 carb, 3 fat
Vanilla Ice Cream/ Chocolate Roll	1/2 cup	270	14	46	4	0	45	340	39	2	4	2 1/2 carb, 3 fat
Vanilla Ice Cream/ Devil's Food	2/3 cup	340	19	50	9	0	60	220	39	1	5	2 1/2 carb, 3 1/2 fat
LOW FAT ICE CREAM												
Espresso 'n Cream	1/2 cup	180	4	20	1.5	0	10	120	32	1	5	2 carb, 1 fat
NO SUGAR ADDED ICE CREAM												
✓Berries 'n Banana Low Fat	1/2 cup	110	2	16	1	0	10	125	25	1	5	1 1/2 carb, 1/2 fat

Carmel Turtle Low Fat	1/2 cup	160	4	22	3	0	10	130	37	0	5	2 carb, 1 fat
✔Chocolate Chip Low Fat	1/2 cup	170	4.5	23	3.5	0	10	110	30	1	4	2 carb, 1 fat
✔Chocolate Chocolate Chip	1/2 cup	150	4.5	27	3.5	0	10	140	30	1	6	2 carb, 1 fat
Chocolate Cookie Low Fat	1/2 cup	160	5	28	2	0.5	10	190	34	1	6	2 carb, 1 fat
Mad About Chocolate Low Fat	1/2 cup	160	5	28	3.5	0	10	125	36	1	5	2 carb, 1 fat
✔Pineapple Coconut Low Fat	1/2 cup	150	2	12	1.5	0	10	105	27	0	4	1 1/2 carb, 1/2 fat
Tin Roof Sundae Low Fat	1/2 cup	190	3	14	1.5	0	10	105	34	1	4	2 carb, 1/2 fat

NO SUGAR ADDED SOFT SERVE YOGURT

✔Truly Free Butter Pecan	1/2 cup	90	0	0	0	0	5	90	17	1	4	1 carb
✔Truly Free Café Mocha	1/2 cup	90	0	0	0	0	5	85	18	1	4	1 carb
✔Truly Free Chocolate	1/2 cup	80	0	0	0	0	0	80	15	0	4	1 carb
✔Truly Free Strawberry	1/2 cup	90	0	0	0	0	5	85	17	1	4	1 carb
✔Truly Free Vanilla	1/2 cup	90	0	0	0	0	0	85	17	1	4	1 carb

✔ = Healthiest Bets

(Continued)

	Amount	Cal.	Fat (g)	% Cal. Fat	Sat. Fat (g)	Trans Fat (g)	Chol. (mg)	Sod. (mg)	Carb. (g)	Fiber (g)	Pro. (g)	Servings/Exchanges
REGULAR DELUXE ICE CREAMS												
Banana Nut	1/2 cup	260	16	55	7	0	45	75	27	1	5	1 1/2 carb, 3 fat
Bananas 'n Strawberry	1/2 cup	220	9	36	6	0	35	70	34	0	3	2 carb, 2 fat
Baseball Nut	1/2 cup	270	14	46	8	0	45	100	32	0	5	2 carb, 2 fat
Black Walnut	1/2 cup	280	19	61	9	0	50	90	25	1	6	1 1/2 carb, 3 1/2 fat
Blueberry Cheesecake	1/2 cup	270	14	46	8	0.5	55	125	32	0	5	2 carb, 3 fat
Boston Cream Pie	1/2 cup	280	14	45	8	1	70	135	36	0	5	2 carb, 3 fat
Candy Cookie Commotion	1/2 cup	300	16	48	9	0	45	150	36	1	5	2 carb, 3 fat
Cherries Jubilee	1/2 cup	240	12	45	7	0	45	80	30	1	6	2 carb, 2 1/2 fat
Chocoholic's Resolution	1/2 cup	300	16	48	9	0	45	130	38	0	5	2 1/2 carb, 3 fat
Chocolate	1/2 cup	260	14	48	9	0	50	130	33	0	5	2 carb, 3 fat

Chocolate Almond	1/2 cup	300	18	54	9	0	45	120	32	1	7	2 carb, 3 1/2 fat
Chocolate Chip	1/2 cup	270	16	53	10	0	55	95	28	1	5	2 carb, 3 fat
Chocolate Chip Cookie Dough	1/2 cup	290	15	46	9	1	55	130	36	1	5	2 carb, 3 fat
Chocolate Éclair	1/2 cup	300	17	51	11	0	60	130	35	0	5	2 carb, 3 fat
Chocolate Fudge	1/2 cup	270	15	50	10	0	50	140	35	0	4	2 carb, 3 fat
Chocolate Mousse Crossing	1/2 cup	270	15	50	9	0	50	115	32	0	5	2 carb, 3 fat
Chocolate Mousse Royale	1/2 cup	310	16	46	12	0	40	140	38	1	6	2 1/2 carb, 3 1/2 fat
Chocolate Ribbon	1/2 cup	240	12	45	8	0	45	85	31	0	4	2 carb, 2 1/2 fat
Crème Brulee	1/2 cup	280	11	35	7	0	80	115	41	0	4	3 carb, 2 fat
Egg Nog	1/2 cup	250	13	46	8	0	70	90	31	0	5	2 carb, 2 1/2 fat
French Vanilla	1/2 cup	280	18	57	11	0.5	120	85	26	0	4	1 1/2 carb, 3 1/2 fat

(Continued)

✔ = Healthiest Bets

REGULAR DELUXE ICE CREAMS *(Continued)*	Amount	Cal.	Fat (g)	% Cal. Fat	Sat. Fat (g)	Trans Fat (g)	Chol. (mg)	Sod. (mg)	Carb. (g)	Fiber (g)	Pro. (g)	Servings/Exchanges
Fudge Brownie	1/2 cup	300	19	57	11	0	45	140	35	1	5	2 carb, 4 fat
German Chocolate Cake	1/2 cup	300	16	48	9	0	45	150	36	1	5	2 carb, 3 fat
Gold Metal Ribbon	1/2 cup	260	13	45	8	0	45	150	34	0	5	2 carb, 2 1/2 fat
Here Comes the Fudge	1/2 cup	280	12	38	7	1	45	120	39	1	4	2 1/2 carb, 2 1/2 fat
Honest to Goodnuts	1/2 cup	300	14	42	8	0	40	135	38	0	5	2 1/2 carb, 3 fat
Hunka Chunka Chip	1/2 cup	300	15	45	8	1	45	170	37	0	5	2 1/2 carb, 3 fat
Jamoca	1/2 cup	240	13	48	9	0	55	90	26	0	5	2 carb, 3 fat
Jamoca Almond	1/2 cup	270	15	50	7	0	40	80	31	1	6	2 carb, 3 fat
Lemon Custard	1/2 cup	260	13	45	8	0	75	105	30	0	5	2 carb, 2 1/2 fat
Love Potion #31	1/2 cup	270	14	46	9	0	45	90	34	1	4	2 carb, 3 fat
Macadamia Nuts 'n Cream	1/2 cup	290	20	62	9	0	50	85	25	1	5	2 carb, 4 fat
Mint Chocolate Chip	1/2 cup	270	16	53	10	0	55	95	28	1	5	2 carb, 3 fat

Mississippi Mudd	1/2 cup	270	13	43	8	0	45	150	38	1	4	2 1/2 carb, 2 1/2 fat
New York Cheesecake	1/2 cup	280	16	51	10	0	50	135	31	0	5	2 carb, 3 fat
Nutty Coconut	1/2 cup	300	20	60	9	0	45	90	28	1	6	2 carb, 4 fat
Old Fashion Butter Pecan	1/2 cup	280	18	57	9	0	50	95	24	1	5	1 1/2 carb, 3 1/2 fat
Oregon Blackberry	1/2 cup	240	12	45	8	0	50	85	28	0	4	2 carb, 2 1/2 fat
Oreo Cookies 'n Cream	1/2 cup	280	15	48	8	1	50	150	32	1	5	2 carb, 3 fat
Original Cinn	1/2 cup	290	13	40	8	0	45	130	39	0	4	2 1/2 carb, 2 1/2 fat
Peanut Butter 'n Chocolate	1/2 cup	320	20	56	9	0	45	180	31	1	7	2 carb, 4 fat
Peppermint	1/2 cup	270	14	46	9	0	50	85	32	0	4	2 carb, 3 fat
Pink Bubblegum	1/2 cup	260	12	41	8	0	50	80	36	0	4	2 carb, 2 1/2 fat
Pistachio Almond	1/2 cup	290	19	58	9	0	50	85	25	1	7	1 1/2 carb, 4 fat
Pralines 'n Cream	1/2 cup	270	14	46	8	0	45	170	34	0	4	2 carb, 3 fat
Pumpkin Pie	1/2 cup	230	12	46	7	0	45	90	29	0	4	2 carb, 2 1/2 fat

(Continued)

✔ = Healthiest Bets

REGULAR DELUXE ICE CREAMS *(Continued)*	Amount	Cal.	Fat (g)	% Cal. Fat	Sat. Fat (g)	Trans Fat (g)	Chol. (mg)	Sod. (mg)	Carb. (g)	Fiber (g)	Pro. (g)	Servings/Exchanges
Quarterback Crunch	1/2 cup	300	17	51	12	0	45	150	34	0	4	3 carb, 3 fat
Reese's Peanut Butter Cup	1/2 cup	300	18	54	10	0	50	130	31	0	6	2 carb, 3 fat
Rocky Road	1/2 cup	290	15	46	8	0	45	120	36	1	5	2 carb, 3 fat
Strawberry Cheesecake	1/2 cup	270	14	46	9	0.5	55	115	32	0	5	2 carb, 2 1/2 fat
Strawberry Shortcake	1/2 cup	280	14	45	9	0	45	130	34	0	4	2 carb, 3 fat
Tax Crunch	1/2 cup	300	18	54	8	0	45	135	32	1	5	2 carb, 3 fat
Tiramisu	1/2 cup	260	13	45	8	0	60	120	32	0	5	2 carb, 2 1/2 fat
Trick Oreo Treat	1/2 cup	300	16	48	9	0	45	150	36	1	5	2 carb, 3 fat
True Blue Ginger	1/2 cup	270	13	43	8	0	50	140	33	0	4	2 carb, 2 1/2 fat
Truffle in Paradise	1/2 cup	330	21	57	12	0	50	75	34	1	5	2 carb, 4 fat
Vanilla	1/2 cup	260	16	55	10	0.5	65	70	26	0	4	1 1/2 carb, 3 fat
Very Berry Strawberry	1/2 cup	220	11	45	7	0	40	70	28	0	4	2 carb, 2 fat

Winter White Chocolate	1/2 cup	270	14	46	10	0	40	95	32	1	4	2 carb, 3 fat
World Class Chocolate	1/2 cup	270	15	50	8	0.5	45	115	33	0	5	2 carb, 3 fat

SHAKES

Chocolate Shake w/ Chocolate Ice Cream	24 oz	990	40	36	25	1	135	440	149	1	20	1 1/2 carb, 9 fat
Chocolate Shake w/ Vanilla Ice Cream	16 oz	690	33	43	21	0	130	210	85	0	13	5 carb, 6 1/2 fat
Chocolate w/ Chocolate Ice Cream	16 oz	620	30	43	18	1	105	300	81	1	15	5 carb, 6 fat
Chocolate w/ Vanilla Ice Cream	24 oz	1000	45	40	28	0	175	290	133	0	19	9 carb, 9 fat
Espresso Shake	24 oz	790	45	51	28	0	175	300	80	0	19	5 carb, 9 fat
Vanilla Shake	16 oz	680	33	43	21	0	130	380	81	0	13	5 carb, 6 1/2 fat
Vanilla Shake	24 oz	980	45	41	28	0	175	640	125	0	19	8 carb, 9 fat

(Continued)

✔ = Healthiest Bets

SHERBETS & ICES

	Amount	Cal.	Fat (g)	% Cal. Fat	Sat. Fat (g)	Trans Fat (g)	Chol. (mg)	Sod. (mg)	Carb. (g)	Fiber (g)	Pro. (g)	Servings/Exchanges
Blue Raspberry Sherbet	1/2 cup	160	2	11	1.5	0	10	40	34	0	1	2 carb
Daiquiri Ice	1/2 cup	130	0	0	0	0	0	15	34	0	0	2 carb
Margarita Ice	1/2 cup	130	0	0	0	0	0	15	34	0	0	2 carb
Orange Sherbet	1/2 cup	160	2	11	1.5	0	10	40	34	0	1	2 carb
Pineapple Ice/Sorbet	1/2 cup	140	0	0	0	0	0	10	36	0	0	2 carb
Rainbow Sherbet	1/2 cup	160	2	11	1.5	0	10	40	34	0	1	2 carb
Red Raspberry Sherbet	1/2 cup	160	2	11	1.5	0	10	40	36	0	1	2 carb
Rock 'n Pop Swirl Sherbet	1/2 cup	190	4	18	3	0	10	45	37	0	1	2 carb, 1 fat
Watermelon Ice	1/2 cup	130	0	0	0	0	0	15	34	0	0	2 carb
Wild 'n Reckless Spirit Sherbet	1/2 cup	160	2	11	1.5	0	10	40	34	0	1	2 carb

SUNDAES

2 Scoop Hot Fudge Sundae	1	530	29	49	19	0	85	200	62	0	8	4 carb, 6 fat
3 Scoop Hot Fudge Sundae	1	750	41	49	27	0	125	280	86	0	11	5 1/2 carb, 8 fat
Banana Royale	1	630	27	38	16	0	85	250	91	5	9	6 carb, 5 1/2 fat
Banana Split	1	1030	39	34	23	0	135	190	168	7	12	11 carb, 4 fat

✔ = Healthiest Bets

Burger King

www.burgerking.com

Light & Lean Choice

1 Fire-Grilled Chicken Caesar Salad
Tomato Balsamic Vinaigrette (2 T)
Low-Fat Milk (8 oz)
1 Mott's Strawberry Applesauce

Calories	437	Cholesterol (mg)	62
Fat (g)	14	Sodium (mg)	1,767
% calories from fat	29	Carbohydrate (g)	53
Saturated fat (g)	6	Fiber (g)	1
Trans fat (g)	0	Protein (g)	33

Exchanges: 1 carb, 1 fruit, 2 lean meat, 3 fat

Healthy & Hearty Choice

1 Whopper Jr. with Cheese
French Fries (small order)
1 Mott's Strawberry Applesauce

Calories	670	Cholesterol (mg)	50
Fat (g)	28	Sodium (mg)	1,110
% calories from fat	38	Carbohydrate (g)	84
Saturated fat (g)	11	Fiber (g)	4
Trans fat (g)	1	Protein (g)	22

Exchanges: 4 1/2 starch, 1 fruit, 2 medium-fat meat, 2 fat

(Continued)

Burger King

BREAKFAST

	Amount	Cal.	Fat (g)	% Cal. Fat	Sat. Fat (g)	Trans Fat (g)	Chol. (mg)	Sod. (mg)	Carb. (g)	Fiber (g)	Pro. (g)	Servings/Exchanges
Croissan'wich w/ Bacon, Egg & Cheese	1	340	20	52	7	1.5	200	920	26	0	14	1 1/2 starch, 2 high-fat meat, 1 fat
Croissan'wich w/ Egg & Cheese	1	300	17	51	6	1.5	195	700	26	0	12	1 1/2 starch, 1 medium-fat meat, 2 1/2 fat
Croissan'wich w/ Ham, Egg & Cheese	1	340	18	47	6	1.5	210	1470	26	0	17	1 1/2 starch, 2 medium-fat meat, 1 fat
Croissan'wich w/ Sausage and Cheese	1	410	29	63	11	2	45	840	24	1	13	1 1/2 starch, 1 high-fat meat, 4 fat
Croissan'wich w/ Sausage, Egg & Cheese	1	500	36	64	12	2	220	1060	26	1	18	1 1/2 starch, 2 high-fat meat, 4 fat

Item	Serving										Exchanges
Double Croissan'wich w/ Double Bacon	1	430	26	54	11	2	220	1360	27	0	19	1 1/2 starch, 2 high-fat meat, 2 fat
Double Croissan'wich w/ Double Ham	1	420	23	49	9	2	235	2450	27	0	26	1 1/2 starch, 3 lean meat, 3 fat
Double Croissan'wich w/ Double Sausage	1	750	60	72	21	3	260	1630	26	2	28	1 1/2 starch, 3 high-fat meat, 9 fat
Double Croissan'wich w/ Ham & Bacon	1	420	25	53	10	2	225	1910	27	0	23	1 1/2 starch, 3 high-fat meat
Double Croissan'wich w/ Ham & Sausage	1	580	41	63	15	2.5	245	2040	27	1	27	1 1/2 starch, 3 high-fat meat, 3 1/2 fat
Double Croissan'wich w/ Sausage & Bacon	1	590	43	65	16	2.5	240	1490	27	1	24	1 1/2 starch, 3 high-fat meat, 3 1/2 fat
French Toast Sticks	5 sticks	390	20	46	4.5	4.5	0	440	46	2	6	3 starch, 3 1/2 fat
Hash Brown Rounds, large	1 serving	390	25	57	7	7	0	760	38	4	3	2 1/2 starch, 4 fat

(Continued)

✔ = Healthiest Bets

BREAKFAST *(Continued)*	Amount	Cal.	Fat (g)	% Cal. Fat	Sat. Fat (g)	Trans Fat (g)	Chol. (mg)	Sod. (mg)	Carb. (g)	Fiber (g)	Pro. (g)	Servings/Exchanges
Hash Brown Rounds, small	1 serving	230	15	58	4	5	0	450	23	2	2	1 1/2 starch, 3 fat
BURGERS												
Original Whopper w/out mayo	1	540	24	40	10	1	75	900	52	4	30	3 1/2 starch, 3 medium-fat meat, 1 1/2 fat
Original Whopper w/ cheese low carb	1	370	28	68	14	1	95	720	5	0	27	4 medium-fat meat, 1 1/2 fat
Original Double Whopper low carb	1	540	40	66	18	2	150	380	3	0	43	6 medium-fat meat, 2 fat
Original Double Whopper w/ cheese low carb	1	630	47	67	23	2	170	810	5	0	48	7 medium-fat meat, 2 1/2 fat
Original Double Whopper w/ cheese w/out mayo	1	900	51	51	24	2	170	1410	53	4	56	3 1/2 starch, 4 medium-fat meat, 2 1/2 fat

Original Double Whopper w/out mayo	1	810	44	48	19	2	150	980	52	4	52	3 1/2 starch, 6 medium-fat meat, 3 fat
✔ Original Whopper Jr. low carb	1	140	10	64	4.5	0	40	140	1	0	11	2 medium-fat meat
✔ Original Whopper Jr. w/ cheese low carb	1	190	14	66	7	0.5	50	360	2	0	14	2 high-fat meat
✔ Original Whopper Jr. w/ cheese w/out mayo	1	350	17	43	8	0.5	50	700	32	2	19	2 starch, 2 medium-fat meat, 1 fat
✔ Original Whopper Jr. w/out mayo	1	310	13	37	5	0.5	40	490	31	2	17	2 starch, 2 medium-fat meat, 1/2 fat
✔ Original Whopper low carb	1	280	20	64	9	1	75	290	3	0	22	3 medium-fat meat, 1 fat
Original Whopper w/ cheese w/out mayo	1	640	31	43	15	1.5	95	1330	53	4	35	3 1/2 starch, 4 medium-fat meat, 1 1/2 fat

CHICKEN & FISH

Big Fish Sandwich	1	630	30	42	5	1.5	55	1340	69	4	23	4 1/2 starch, 2 medium-fat meat, 3 fat

(Continued)

✔ = Healthiest Bets

CHICKEN & FISH *(Continued)*	Amount	Cal.	Fat (g)	% Cal. Fat	Sat. Fat (g)	Trans Fat (g)	Chol. (mg)	Sod. (mg)	Carb. (g)	Fiber (g)	Pro. (g)	Servings/Exchanges
Chicken Tenders	8 pieces	340	19	50	5	3.5	50	840	20	0	22	1 starch, 3 lean meat, 2 fat
✔Chicken Tenders	6 pieces	250	14	50	4	2.5	35	630	15	0	16	1 starch, 2 lean meat, 1 1/2 fat
✔Chicken Tenders	4 pieces	170	9	47	2.5	2	25	420	10	0	11	1/2 starch, 1 lean meat, 2 fat
✔Chicken Tenders	5 pieces	210	12	51	3.5	2.5	30	530	13	0	14	1 starch, 2 lean meat, 1 1/2 fat
Chicken Whopper Sandwich w/ mayo	1	570	25	39	4.5	0	75	1410	48	4	38	3 starch, 4 medium-fat meat, 1 fat
Chicken Whopper Sandwich w/out mayo	1	410	7	15	2	0	60	1280	48	4	38	3 starch, 4 lean meat
Original Chicken Sandwich w/out mayo	1	460	17	33	4.5	2	55	1190	52	3	25	3 1/2 starch, 2 lean meat, 2 fat

Item	Amt	Cal	Fat	%Fat	Sat	Trans	Chol	Sod	Carb	Fib	Pro	Exchanges/Choices
Spicy Big Fish Sandwich	1	630	30	42	5	1.5	55	1490	69	4	23	4 1/2 starch, 2 medium-fat meat, 3 fat
Spicy Big Fish Sandwich w/out tartar sauce	1	480	13	24	2.5	1.5	40	1190	68	4	23	4 1/2 starch, 1 medium-fat meat, 1 fat
Spicy Tender Crisp Chicken Sandwich	1	720	37	46	6	3.5	50	1990	71	6	26	4 1/2 starch, 2 lean meat, 6 fat
Spicy Tender Crisp Chicken Sandwich w/out sauce or mayo	1	570	21	33	3.5	3.5	40	1540	70	6	26	4 1/2 starch, 2 lean meat, 2 1/2 fat
Tender Crisp Chicken Sandwich	1	780	45	51	7	4	55	1730	70	6	27	4 1/2 starch, 2 lean meat, 7 fat
DESSERTS												
Dutch Apple Pie	1	300	13	39	3	3	0	270	45	1	2	3 carb, 2 fat
Hershey's Sundae Pie	1	300	18	54	10	1.5	10	190	31	1	3	2 carb, 3 1/2 fat

✔ = Healthiest Bets

	Amount	Cal.	Fat (g)	% Cal. Fat	Sat. Fat (g)	Trans Fat (g)	Chol. (mg)	Sod. (mg)	Carb. (g)	Fiber (g)	Pro. (g)	Servings/Exchanges
DIPPING SAUCES												
Barbecue	2 T	35	0	0	0	n/a	0	390	9	0	0	1/2 carb
Honey Flavor	2 T	90	0	0	0	n/a	0	0	23	0	0	1 1/2 carb
Honey Mustard	2 T	90	6	60	1	n/a	10	150	9	0	0	1/2 carb
Ranch	2 T	140	15	96	2.5	n/a	5	95	1	0	1	3 fat
✔ Sweet and Sour	2 T	40	0	0	0	n/a	0	65	10	0	0	1/2 carb
Zesty Onion	2 T	150	15	90	2.5	0	15	210	3	0	0	3 fat
FIRE-GRILLED BURGERS												
Bacon Cheeseburger	1	390	20	46	9	0.5	60	990	31	1	22	2 starch, 2 high-fat meat, 1/2 fat
Bacon Double Cheeseburger	1	570	34	53	17	1.5	110	1250	32	2	35	2 starch, 4 high-fat meat

	Serving										Exchanges
✔Cheeseburger	1	350	17	43	8	0.5	50	770	31	1	19	2 starch, 2 medium-fat meat, 1 1/2 fat
Double Cheeseburger	1	530	31	52	15	1.5	100	1030	32	2	32	2 starch, 4 medium-fat meat, 2 fat
Double Hamburger	1	440	23	47	10	1	75	600	30	1	28	2 starch, 3 medium-fat meat, 1 1/2 fat
✔Hamburger	1	310	13	37	5	0.5	40	550	30	1	17	2 starch, 2 medium-fat meat, 1/2 fat
The Angus Bacon and Cheese	1	710	33	41	15	1.5	21	1990	64	3	41	4 starch, 4 medium-fat meat, 2 fat
The Angus Steak Burger	1	570	22	34	8	1	180	1270	62	3	33	4 starch, 3 medium-fat meat, 1 fat

MILK SHAKES

	Serving										Exchanges
Chocolate	medium	600	18	27	11	0	70	470	97	2	10	6 1/2 carb, 3 1/2 fat
Chocolate	small	410	13	28	8	0	50	300	65	0	7	4 carb, 2 1/2 fat

✔ = Healthiest Bets   n/a = not available

(Continued)

MILK SHAKES *(Continued)*	Amount	Cal.	Fat (g)	% Cal. Fat	Sat. Fat (g)	Trans Fat (g)	Chol. (mg)	Sod. (mg)	Carb. (g)	Fiber (g)	Pro. (g)	Servings/Exchanges
Chocolate	large	850	27	28	17	0.5	105	620	133	2	15	9 carb, 5 1/2 fat
Strawberry	medium	590	17	25	11	0	70	300	96	0	9	6 1/2 carb, 3 1/2 fat
Strawberry	large	840	26	27	17	0.5	105	450	131	0	14	9 carb, 5 fat
Strawberry	small	410	13	28	8	0	50	220	64	0	7	4 carb, 2 1/2 fat
Vanilla	small	400	15	33	9	0	60	240	57	0	8	3 1/2 carb, 3 fat
Vanilla	large	800	29	32	19	0.5	120	480	113	0	16	7 1/2 carb, 6 fat
Vanilla	medium	540	20	33	13	1	80	320	76	0	11	5 carb, 4 fat
SALAD DRESSINGS & TOPPINGS												
✔Creamy Garlic Caesar	4 T	130	11	76	2	0	20	710	7	0	2	1/2 starch, 2 fat
✔Fat Free Honey Mustard	4 T	70	0	0	0	0	0	230	18	0	0	1 starch
✔Garden Ranch	4 T	120	10	75	1.5	0	20	610	7	0	0	1/2 starch, 2 fat

Item	Amount	Cal	Fat (g)	% Cal Fat	Sat Fat (g)	Trans Fat (g)	Chol (mg)	Sod (mg)	Carb (g)	Fiber (g)	Prot (g)	Choices/Exchanges
✔ Garlic Parmesan Toast	1 serving	70	3	38	0	0	0	120	9	0	2	1/2 starch, 1/2 fat
✔ Sweet Onion Vinaigrette	4 T	100	8	72	1	0	0	960	8	0	0	1/2 starch, 1 1/2 fat
✔ Tomato Balsamic Vinaigrette	4 T	110	9	73	1	0	0	760	9	0	0	1/2 starch, 1 fat
SALADS												
✔ Fire-Grilled Chicken Caesar Salad w/out dressing or toast	1	190	7	33	3	0	50	900	9	1	25	1/2 carb, 3 lean meat
✔ Fire-Grilled Chicken Garden Salad w/out dressing or toast	1	210	7	30	3	0	50	910	12	2	26	1 starch, 3 lean meat
✔ Fire-Grilled Shrimp Caesar Salad w/out dressing or toast	1	180	10	50	3	0.5	120	880	9	2	20	1/2 starch, 3 lean meat
✔ Fire-Grilled Shrimp Garden Salad w/out dressing or toast	1	200	10	45	3	0.5	120	900	13	3	21	1 starch, 3 lean meat
✔ Side Garden Salad w/out dressing or toast	1	20	0	0	0	0	0	15	4	0	1	1 veg

✔ = Healthiest Bets

(Continued)

SALADS *(Continued)*	Amount	Cal.	Fat (g)	% Cal. Fat	Sat. Fat (g)	Trans Fat (g)	Chol. (mg)	Sod. (mg)	Carb. (g)	Fiber (g)	Pro. (g)	Servings/Exchanges
Tender Crisp Chicken Caesar Salad w/out dressing or toast	1	390	22	50	5	3.5	40	1160	25	4	24	1 starch, 2 veg, 3 medium-fat meat, 1 fat
Tender Crisp Garden Salad w/out dressing or toast	1	410	22	48	5	3.5	40	1170	28	5	25	1 starch, 2 veg, 3 medium-fat meat, 1 1/2 fat
SIDE ORDERS												
Bacon for Whopper Sandwiches	1 strip	15	1	60	0	0	5	70	0	0	1	1/2 fat
French Fries, king salted	1 order	600	30	45	8	8	0	1070	76	6	7	5 starch, 6 fat
French Fries, king unsalted	1 order	600	30	45	8	8	0	620	76	6	7	5 starch, 6 fat
French Fries, large salted	1 order	500	25	45	7	6	0	880	63	5	6	4 starch, 5 fat
French Fries, large unsalted	1 order	500	25	45	7	6	0	510	63	5	6	4 starch, 5 fat

French Fries, medium salted	1 order	360	18	45	5	4.5	0	640	46	4	4	3 starch, 3 1/2 fat
French Fries, medium unsalted	1 order	360	18	45	5	4.5	0	380	46	4	4	3 starch, 3 1/2 fat
French Fries, small salted	1 order	230	11	43	3	3	0	410	29	2	3	2 starch, 2 fat
French Fries, small unsalted	1 order	230	11	43	3	3	0	240	29	2	3	2 starch, 2 fat
✔Mott's Strawberry Flavored Apple Sauce	4 oz	90	0	0	0	0	0	0	23	0	0	1 1/2 fruit
Onion Rings, king	1 order	550	27	44	7	6	5	800	70	5	8	4 1/2 starch, 5 1/2 fat
Onion Rings, large	1 order	480	23	43	6	5	0	690	60	5	7	4 starch, 4 1/2 fat
Onion Rings, medium	1 order	320	16	45	4	3.5	0	460	40	3	4	2 1/2 starch, 3 fat
✔Onion Rings, small	1 order	180	9	45	2	2	0	260	22	2	2	1 1/2 starch, 2 fat

(Continued)

✔ = Healthiest Bets

	Amount	Cal.	Fat (g)	% Cal. Fat	Sat. Fat (g)	Trans Fat (g)	Chol. (mg)	Sod. (mg)	Carb. (g)	Fiber (g)	Pro. (g)	Servings/Exchanges
VEGGIE BURGER												
BK Veggie Burger	1	420	16	34	3	0	10	1090	46	7	23	3 starch, 2 medium-fat meat, 1 fat
✔BK Veggie Burger w/out mayo	1	340	8	21	1.5	0	0	1020	46	7	23	3 starch, 2 lean meat, 1/2 fat

✔ = Healthiest Bets

Domino's Pizza

www.dominos.com

Light & Lean Choice

14" Crunchy Thin Crust Pizza with Sauce, Cheese, Peppers, Onions, and Mushrooms (3 slices)

Calories	450	Cholesterol (mg)	15
Fat (g)	21	Sodium (mg)	1,040
% calories from fat	42	Carbohydrate (g)	69
Saturated fat (g)	6	Fiber (g)	4
Trans fat (g)	0	Protein (g)	15

Exchanges: 3 starch, 3 vegetable, 1 medium-fat meat, 2 fat

Healthy & Hearty Choice

12" Classic Hand-Tossed Crust Pizza with Sauce, Cheese, Peppers, Onions, and Grilled Chicken (4 slices)

Calories	840	Cholesterol (mg)	60
Fat (g)	20	Sodium (mg)	1,280
% calories from fat	21	Carbohydrate (g)	118
Saturated fat (g)	8	Fiber (g)	4
Trans fat (g)	0	Protein (g)	41

Exchanges: 7 starch, 1 vegetable, 3 lean meat, 2 fat

(Continued)

Domino's Pizza

12" CLASSIC HAND-TOSSED

	Amount	Cal.	Fat (g)	% Cal. Fat	Sat. Fat (g)	Trans Fat (g)	Chol. (mg)	Sod. (mg)	Carb. (g)	Fiber (g)	Pro. (g)	Servings/Exchanges
✓American Cheese	1 slice	205	6	26	3	0	10	355	29	1	8	2 starch, 1 fat
✓Anchovies	1 slice	210	6.5	27	1	0	10	310	29	1	9	2 starch, 1 fat
✓Bacon	1 slice	250	9	32	2	0	20	390	29	1	13	2 starch, 2 fat
✓Banana Peppers	1 slice	210	6.5	27	1	0	10	405	29	1	9	2 starch, 1 fat
✓Beef	1 slice	250	9.5	34	2.5	0	20	345	29	1	11	2 starch, 2 fat
✓Black Olives	1 slice	220	7.5	30	1	0	10	340	30	1	9	2 starch, 1 fat
✓Cheddar Cheese	1 slice	195	5.5	25	2.5	0	5	210	29	1	8	2 starch, 1/2 fat
✓Extra Cheese	1 slice	235	8.5	32	2	0	15	360	30	1	11	2 starch, 1 1/2 fat
✓Garlic	1 slice	220	6.5	26	1	0	10	275	30	1	9	2 starch, 1 fat

✔Green Chile Peppers	1 slice	210	6.5	27	1	0	10	275	29	1	9	2 starch, 1 fat
✔Green Olives	1 slice	225	8	32	1	0	10	370	29	1	9	2 starch, 1 fat
✔Green Pepper	1 slice	210	6.5	27	1	0	10	275	29	1	9	2 starch, 1 fat
✔Green Pepper, Onion & Mushroom	1 slice	210	6.5	27	1	0	10	275	29	1	9	2 starch, 1 fat
✔Grilled Chicken	1 slice	230	6.5	25	1	0	20	365	29	1	12	2 starch, 1 very-lean meat, 2 fat
✔Ham	1 slice	220	6.5	26	1	0	15	375	29	1	11	2 starch, 1 fat
✔Ham & Pineapple	1 slice	230	6.5	25	1	0	15	375	31	1	11	2 starch, 1 fat
✔Jalapeño Peppers	1 slice	210	6.5	27	1	0	10	375	29	1	9	2 starch, 1 fat
✔Mushroom	1 slice	210	6.5	27	1	0	10	275	29	1	9	2 starch, 1 fat
✔Onions	1 slice	210	6.5	27	1	0	10	275	30	1	9	2 starch, 1 fat
✔Pepperoni	1 slice	250	10	36	2	0	15	415	29	1	11	2 starch, 2 fat
Pepperoni & Sausage	1 slice	295	13.5	41	3.5	0	20	545	30	1	13	2 starch, 3 fat

✔ = Healthiest Bets

(Continued)

12" CLASSIC HAND-TOSSED (Continued)	Amount	Cal.	Fat (g)	% Cal. Fat	Sat. Fat (g)	Trans Fat (g)	Chol. (mg)	Sod. (mg)	Carb. (g)	Fiber (g)	Pro. (g)	Servings/Exchanges
✔ Philly Steak	1 slice	220	6.5	26	1	0	15	335	29	1	11	2 starch, 1 fat
✔ Pineapple	1 slice	220	6.5	26	1	0	10	275	31	1	9	2 starch, 1 fat
✔ Provolone Cheese	1 slice	210	6.5	27	1	0	10	275	29	1	9	2 starch, 1 fat
Sausage	1 slice	255	10	35	2.5	0	15	405	30	1	11	2 starch, 2 fat
✔ Tomatoes	1 slice	210	6.5	27	1	0	10	275	30	1	9	2 starch, 1 fat
12" CRUNCHY THIN CRUST												
✔ American Cheese	1 slice	125	6.5	46	2.5	0	10	260	13	1	4	1 starch, 1 fat
✔ Anchovies	1 slice	130	7	48	0.5	0	10	215	13	1	5	1 starch, 1 fat
✔ Bacon	1 slice	170	9.5	50	1.5	0	20	295	13	1	9	1 starch, 2 fat
✔ Banana Peppers	1 slice	130	7	48	0.5	0	10	310	13	1	5	1 starch, 1 fat
✔ Beef	1 slice	170	10	52	2	0	20	250	13	1	7	1 starch, 2 fat
✔ Black Olives	1 slice	140	8	51	0.5	0	10	245	14	1	5	1 starch, 1 fat

✔Cheddar Cheese	1 slice	115	6	46	2	0	5	115	13	1	4	1 starch, 1/2 fat
✔Extra Cheese	1 slice	155	9	52	1.5	0	15	265	14	1	7	1 starch, 1 1/2 fat
✔Garlic	1 slice	140	7	45	0.5	0	10	180	14	1	5	1 starch, 1 fat
✔Green Chile Peppers	1 slice	130	7	48	0.5	0	10	180	13	1	5	1 starch, 1 fat
✔Green Olives	1 slice	145	8.5	52	0.5	0	10	275	13	1	5	1 starch, 1 fat
✔Green Pepper	1 slice	130	7	48	0.5	0	10	180	13	1	5	1 starch, 1 fat
✔Green Pepper, Onion & Mushroom	1 slice	130	7	48	0.5	0	10	180	13	1	5	1 starch, 1 fat
✔Grilled Chicken	1 slice	150	7	42	0.5	0	20	270	13	1	8	1 starch, 1 very lean meat, 1 fat
✔Ham	1 slice	140	7	45	0.5	0	15	280	13	1	7	1 starch, 1 fat
✔Ham & Pineapple	1 slice	130	7	48	0.5	0	10	180	13	1	5	1 starch, 1 fat
✔Jalapeño Peppers	1 slice	130	7	48	0.5	0	10	280	13	1	5	1 starch, 1 fat
✔Mushroom	1 slice	130	7	48	0.5	0	10	180	13	1	5	1 starch, 1 fat

✔ = Healthiest Bets

(Continued)

12" CRISPY THIN CRUST *(Continued)*	Amount	Cal.	Fat (g)	% Cal. Fat	Sat. Fat (g)	Trans Fat (g)	Chol. (mg)	Sod. (mg)	Carb. (g)	Fiber (g)	Pro. (g)	Servings/Exchanges
✔Onions	1 slice	130	7	48	0.5	0	10	180	14	1	5	1 starch, 1 fat
✔Pepperoni	1 slice	170	10.5	55	1.5	0	15	320	13	1	7	1 starch, 2 fat
Pepperoni & Sausage	1 slice	215	14	58	3	0	20	450	14	1	9	1 starch, 3 fat
✔Philly Steak	1 slice	140	7	45	0.5	0	15	240	13	1	7	1 starch, 1 fat
✔Pineapple	1 slice	140	7	45	0.5	0	10	180	15	1	5	1 starch, 1 fat
✔Provolone Cheese	1 slice	130	7	48	0.5	0	10	180	13	1	5	1 starch, 1 fat
Sausage	1 slice	175	10.5	54	2	0	15	310	14	1	7	1 starch, 2 fat
✔Tomatoes	1 slice	130	7	48	0.5	0	10	180	14	1	5	1 starch, 1 fat
12" FEAST PIZZAS CLASSIC HAND-TOSSED												
America's Favorite	1 slice	290	13	40	5	0	20	560	32	2	12	2 starch, 1 high-fat meat, 1 fat

Bacon Cheeseburger	1 slice	300	14	42	6	0	30	500	31	2	15	2 starch, 1 high-fat meat, 1 fat
Barbecue	1 slice	290	11	34	5	0	20	470	36	1	13	2 starch, 1 high-fat meat, 1 fat
Deluxe	1 slice	260	11	38	4.5	0	15	490	32	2	11	2 starch, 1 high-fat meat, 1 fat
Extravaganzza	1 slice	320	15	42	6	0	30	700	33	2	15	2 starch, 1 high-fat meat, 1 fat
✔ Hawaiian	1 slice	250	9	32	4	0	15	500	33	2	12	2 starch, 1 high-fat meat
Meatzza	1 slice	310	14	40	6	0	30	670	32	2	14	2 starch, 1 high-fat meat, 1 fat
Pepperoni	1 slice	290	14	43	6	0	25	640	32	2	13	2 starch, 1 high-fat meat, 1 fat
Philly Cheese	1 slice	260	10	34	5	0	20	470	29	1	13	2 starch, 1 high-fat meat, 1/2 fat

✔ = Healthiest Bets

(Continued)

12" FEAST PIZZA CLASSIC HAND-TOSSED (Continued)

12" FEAST PIZZA CLASSIC HAND-TOSSED (Continued)	Amount	Cal.	Fat (g)	% Cal. Fat	Sat. Fat (g)	Trans Fat (g)	Chol. (mg)	Sod. (mg)	Carb. (g)	Fiber (g)	Pro. (g)	Servings/Exchanges
✔Vegi	1 slice	240	9	33	4	0	15	450	32	2	11	2 starch, 1 high-fat meat

12" FEAST PIZZAS CRUNCHY THIN CRUST

12" FEAST PIZZAS CRUNCHY THIN CRUST	Amount	Cal.	Fat (g)	% Cal. Fat	Sat. Fat (g)	Trans Fat (g)	Chol. (mg)	Sod. (mg)	Carb. (g)	Fiber (g)	Pro. (g)	Servings/Exchanges
America's Favorite	1 slice	210	13	55	5	0	20	465	16	2	8	1 starch, 1 high-fat meat, 1 fat
Bacon Cheeseburger	1 slice	220	14	57	6	0	30	405	15	2	11	1 starch, 1 high-fat meat, 1 fat
Barbecue	1 slice	210	11	47	5	0	20	375	20	1	9	1 starch, 1 high-fat meat, 1 fat
Deluxe	1 slice	180	11	55	4.5	0	15	395	16	2	7	1 starch, 1 high-fat meat, 1 fat
Extravaganzza	1 slice	240	15	56	6	0	30	605	17	2	11	1 starch, 1 high-fat meat, 1 1/2 fat
✔Hawaiian	1 slice	170	9	47	4	0	15	405	17	2	8	1 starch, 1 high-fat meat

Meatzza	1 slice	230	14	54	6	0	30	575	16	2	10	1 starch, 1 high-fat meat, 1 fat
Pepperoni	1 slice	210	14	60	6	0	25	545	16	2	9	1 starch, 1 high-fat meat, 1 fat
✔Philly Cheese	1 slice	180	10	50	5	0	20	375	13	1	9	1 starch, 1 high-fat meat, 1/2 fat
✔Vegi	1 slice	160	9	50	4	0	15	355	16	2	7	1 starch, 1 high-fat meat

12" FEAST PIZZAS ULTIMATE DEEP DISH

America's Favorite	1 slice	290	16	49	5	0	20	700	28	4	10	2 starch, 1 high-fat meat, 1 1/2 fat
Bacon Cheeseburger	1 slice	300	17	51	6	0	30	640	27	4	13	2 starch, 1 high-fat meat, 2 fat
Barbecue	1 slice	290	14	43	5	0	20	610	32	3	11	2 starch, 1 high-fat meat, 1 1/2 fat

(*Continued*)

✔ = Healthiest Bets

12" FEAST PIZZA ULTIMATE DEEP DISH *(Continued)*	Amount	Cal.	Fat (g)	% Cal. Fat	Sat. Fat (g)	Trans Fat (g)	Chol. (mg)	Sod. (mg)	Carb. (g)	Fiber (g)	Pro. (g)	Servings/Exchanges
Deluxe	1 slice	260	14	48	4.5	0	15	630	28	4	9	2 starch, 1 high-fat meat, 1 1/2 fat
Extravaganzza	1 slice	320	18	50	6	0	30	840	29	4	13	2 starch, 1 high-fat meat, 2 fat
Hawaiian	1 slice	250	12	43	4	0	15	640	29	4	10	2 starch, 1 high-fat meat, 1 fat
Meatzza	1 slice	310	17	49	6	0	30	810	28	4	12	2 starch, 1 high-fat meat, 2 fat
Pepperoni	1 slice	290	17	52	6	0	25	780	28	4	11	2 starch, 1 high-fat meat, 2 fat
Philly Cheese	1 slice	260	13	45	5	0	20	610	25	3	11	2 starch, 1 high-fat meat, 1 fat
Vegi	1 slice	240	12	45	4	0	15	590	28	4	9	2 starch, 1 high-fat meat, 1 fat

12" ULTIMATE DEEP DISH

✔ American Cheese	1 slice	205	9	39	3	0	10	495	25	3	6 1 1/2 starch, 2 fat
Anchovies	1 slice	225	11	44	3.5	0	10	560	27	3	8 1 1/2 starch, 2 fat
Bacon	1 slice	265	13.5	45	4.5	0	20	640	27	6	12 1 1/2 starch, 3 fat
Banana Peppers	1 slice	225	11	44	3.5	0	10	655	27	48	8 1 1/2 starch, 2 fat
Beef	1 slice	265	14	47	5	0	20	595	27	384	10 1 1/2 starch, 3 fat
Black Olives	1 slice	235	12	45	3.5	0	10	590	28	384	8 1 1/2 starch, 2 fat
✔ Cheddar Cheese	1 slice	195	8.5	39	2.5	0	5	350	25	3	6 1 1/2 starch, 1 1/2 fat
Cheese	1 slice	225	11	44	3.5	0	10	525	27	3	8 1 1/2 starch, 2 fat
Garlic	1 slice	235	11	42	3.5	0	10	525	28	96	8 1 1/2 starch, 2 fat
Green Chile Peppers	1 slice	225	11	44	3.5	0	10	525	27	192	8 1 1/2 starch, 2 fat
Green Olives	1 slice	240	12.5	46	3.5	0	10	620	27	384	8 1 1/2 starch, 2 fat
Green Pepper	1 slice	225	11	44	3.5	0	10	525	27	384	8 1 1/2 starch, 2 fat

✔ = Healthiest Bets

(Continued)

12" ULTIMATE DEEP DISH *(Continued)*	Amount	Cal.	Fat (g)	% Cal. Fat	Sat. Fat (g)	Trans Fat (g)	Chol. (mg)	Sod. (mg)	Carb. (g)	Fiber (g)	Pro. (g)	Servings/Exchanges
Green Pepper, Onion & Mushroom	1 slice	225	11	44	3.5	0	10	525	28	384	8	1 1/2 starch, 2 fat
Grilled Chicken	1 slice	245	11	40	3.5	0	20	615	27	12	11	1 1/2 starch, 1 very-lean meat, 2 fat
Ham	1 slice	235	11	42	3.5	0	15	625	27	384	10	1 1/2 starch, 2 fat
Ham & Pineapple	1 slice	245	11	40	3.5	0	15	625	29	384	10	1 1/2 starch, 2 fat
Jalapeño Peppers	1 slice	225	11	44	3.5	0	10	625	27	384	8	1 1/2 starch, 2 fat
Mushroom	1 slice	225	11	44	3.5	0	10	525	27	384	8	1 1/2 starch, 2 fat
Onions	1 slice	225	11	44	3.5	0	10	525	28	384	8	1 1/2 starch, 2 fat
Pepperoni	1 slice	265	14.5	49	4.5	0	15	665	27	384	10	1 1/2 starch, 3 fat
Pepperoni & Sausage	1 slice	310	18	52	6	0	20	795	28	384	12	1 1/2 starch, 4 fat
Philly Steak	1 slice	235	11	42	3.5	0	15	585	27	24	10	1 1/2 starch, 2 fat

Pineapple	1 slice	235	11	42	3.5	0	10	525	29	384	8	1 1/2 starch, 2 fat
✔ Provolone Cheese	1 slice	210	9.5	40	1	0	10	415	25	3	7	1 1/2 starch, 2 fat
Sausage	1 slice	270	14.5	48	5	0	15	655	28	384	10	1 1/2 starch, 3 fat
Tomatoes	1 slice	225	11	44	3.5	0	10	525	28	384	8	1 1/2 starch, 2 fat

14" CLASSIC HAND-TOSSED

✔ American Cheese	1 slice	275	8	26	3.5	0	10	450	40	3	10	3 starch, 2 fat
Anchovies	1 slice	290	9	27	3.5	0	5	505	42	3	12	3 starch, 2 fat
Bacon	1 slice	350	13	33	5	0	20	640	42	3	18	3 starch, 1 medium fat meat, 2 fat
Banana Peppers	1 slice	290	9	27	3.5	0	5	650	43	3	12	3 starch, 2 fat
✔ Beef	1 slice	280	8.5	27	3	0	10	330	40	3	11	3 starch, 3 fat
Black Olives	1 slice	300	9.5	28	3.5	0	5	530	43	3	12	3 starch, 2 fat
✔ Cheddar Cheese	1 slice	265	7	23	3	0	10	285	40	3	10	3 starch, 2 fat

✔ = Healthiest Bets

(Continued)

14" CLASSIC HAND-TOSSED *(Continued)*/ Amount	Cal.	Fat (g)	% Cal. Fat	Sat. Fat (g)	Trans Fat (g)	Chol. (mg)	Sod. (mg)	Carb. (g)	Fiber (g)	Pro. (g)	Servings/Exchanges
✔Cheese	1 slice	290	9	27	3.5	0	5	470	42	3	12	3 starch, 2 fat
Extra Cheese	1 slice	320	11.5	32	5	0	10	590	43	3	14	3 starch, 3 fat
✔Garlic	1 slice	305	9	26	3.5	0	5	470	43	3	12	3 starch, 2 fat
✔Green Chile Peppers	1 slice	290	9	27	3.5	0	5	470	42	3	12	3 starch, 2 fat
✔Green Olives	1 slice	250	6	21	1	0	0	255	41	3	8	3 starch, 2 fat
✔Green Pepper	1 slice	290	9	27	3.5	0	5	470	42	3	12	3 starch, 2 fat
✔Green Pepper, Onion & Mushroom	1 slice	290	9	27	3.5	0	5	470	44	3	12	3 starch, 2 fat
Grilled Chicken	1 slice	315	9.5	27	3.5	0	20	600	42	3	17	3 starch, 1 very-lean meat, 2 fat
Ham	1 slice	305	9.5	28	3.5	0	5	610	42	3	14	3 starch, 2 fat
Ham & Pineapple	1 slice	320	9.5	26	3.5	0	5	610	45	3	14	3 starch, 3 fat

	Serving	Cal.	Fat (g)		Sat. Fat	Trans Fat	Chol.	Sod.	Carb.	Fiber	Pro.	Exchanges
Jalapeño Peppers	1 slice	290	9	27	3.5	0	5	605	42	3	12	3 starch, 2 fat
✔ Mushroom	1 slice	290	9	27	3.5	0	5	470	43	3	12	3 starch, 2 fat
✔ Onion	1 slice	290	9	27	3.5	0	5	470	43	3	12	3 starch, 2 fat
Pepperoni	1 slice	340	13.5	35	5	0	15	660	42	3	14	3 starch, 3 fat
Pepperoni & Sausage	1 slice	400	19	42	7	0	25	850	44	4	16	3 starch, 1 high-fat meat, 2 fat
Philly Steak	1 slice	305	9.5	28	3.5	0	10	555	42	3	14	3 starch, 2 fat
✔ Pineapple	1 slice	305	9	26	3.5	0	5	470	45	3	12	3 starch, 2 fat
✔ Provolone Cheese	1 slice	290	8.5	26	4	0	10	390	40	3	13	3 starch, 2 fat
Sausage	1 slice	350	14.5	37	5.5	0	15	660	44	4	14	3 starch, 3 fat
✔ Tomatoes	1 slice	290	9	27	3.5	0	5	470	43	3	12	3 starch, 2 fat
14" CRUNCHY THIN CRUST												
✔ American Cheese	1 slice	165	8.5	46	3	0	10	500	18	2	5	1 starch, 1 1/2 fat

(Continued)

✔ = Healthiest Bets

14" CRUNCHY THIN CRUST *(Continued)*	Amount	Cal.	Fat (g)	% Cal. Fat	Sat. Fat (g)	Trans Fat (g)	Chol. (mg)	Sod. (mg)	Carb. (g)	Fiber (g)	Pro. (g)	Servings/Exchanges
Anchovies	1 slice	180	9.5	47	3	0	5	555	20	2	7	1 starch, 1 medium-fat meat, 1 fat
Bacon	1 slice	240	13.5	50	4.5	0	20	690	20	2	13	1 starch, 2 medium-fat meat, 1 fat
✔Banana Peppers	1 slice	180	9.5	47	3	0	5	700	21	2	7	1 starch, 1 medium-fat meat, 1 fat
Beef	1 slice	230	14	54	5	0	15	620	20	2	10	1 starch, 1 medium-fat meat, 2 fat
Black Olives	1 slice	190	10	47	3	0	5	580	21	2	7	1 starch, 1 medium-fat meat, 1 fat
✔Cheddar Cheese	1 slice	155	7.5	43	2.5	0	10	335	18	2	5	1 starch, 2 fat
Cheese	1 slice	180	9.5	47	3	0	5	520	20	2	7	1 starch, 1 medium-fat meat, 1 fat

	Amount										Exchanges
Extra Cheese	1 slice	210	12	51	4.5	0	10	640	21	2	9	1 starch, 1 medium-fat meat, 1 fat
✔Garlic	1 slice	195	9.5	43	3	0	5	520	21	2	7	1 starch, 1 medium-fat meat, 1 fat
✔Green Chile Peppers	1 slice	180	9.5	47	3	0	5	520	20	2	7	1 starch, 1 medium-fat meat, 1 fat
Green Olives	1 slice	200	11.5	51	3	0	5	645	21	2	7	1 starch, 1 medium-fat meat, 1 fat
✔Green Pepper	1 slice	180	9.5	47	3	0	5	520	21	2	7	1 starch, 1 medium-fat meat, 1 fat
✔Green Pepper, Onion & Mushroom	1 slice	180	9.5	47	3	0	5	520	23	2	7	1 starch, 1 medium-fat meat, 1 fat
✔Grilled Chicken	1 slice	205	10	43	3	0	20	650	20	2	12	1 starch, 2 medium-fat meat
✔Ham	1 slice	195	10	46	3	0	5	660	20	2	9	1 starch, 1 medium-fat meat, 1 fat

✔ = Healthiest Bets

(Continued)

14" CRUNCHY THIN CRUST	Amount	Cal.	Fat (g)	% Cal. Fat	Sat. Fat (g)	Trans Fat (g)	Chol. (mg)	Sod. (mg)	Carb. (g)	Fiber (g)	Pro. (g)	Servings/Exchanges
Ham & Pineapple	1 slice	210	10	42	3	0	5	660	23	2	9	1 starch, 1 medium-fat meat, 1 fat
Jalapeño Peppers	1 slice	180	9.5	47	3	0	5	655	20	2	7	1 starch, 1 medium-fat meat, 1 fat
✔Mushroom	1 slice	180	9.5	47	3	0	5	520	21	2	7	1 starch, 1 medium-fat meat, 1 fat
✔Onion	1 slice	180	9.5	47	3	0	5	520	21	2	7	1 starch, 1 medium-fat meat, 1 fat
Pepperoni	1 slice	230	14	54	4.5	0	15	710	20	2	9	1 starch, 1 medium-fat meat, 2 fat
Pepperoni & Sausage	1 slice	290	19.5	60	6.5	0	25	900	22	3	11	1 starch, 2 medium-fat meat, 2 fat
Philly Steak	1 slice	195	10	46	3	0	10	605	20	2	9	1 starch, 1 medium-fat meat, 1 fat

	Amount	Cal.	Fat (g)	% Fat Cal.	Sat. Fat (g)	Trans Fat (g)	Chol. (mg)	Sodium (mg)	Carb. (g)	Fiber (g)	Prot. (g)	Servings/Exchanges
✔Pineapple	1 slice	195	9.5	43	3	0	5	520	23	2	7	1 starch, 1 medium-fat meat, 1 fat
✔Provolone Cheese	1 slice	180	9	45	3.5	0	10	440	18	2	8	1 starch, 2 fat
Sausage	1 slice	240	15	56	5	0	15	710	22	3	9	1 starch, 1 medium-fat meat, 2 fat
✔Tomatoes	1 slice	180	9.5	47	3	0	5	520	20	2	7	1 starch, 1 medium-fat meat, 1 fat
14" FEAST PIZZAS CLASSIC HAND-TOSSED												
America's Favorite	1 slice	390	18	41	7	0	30	790	44	3	17	3 starch, 1 high-fat meat, 2 fat
Bacon Cheeseburger	1 slice	420	19	40	8	0	40	700	42	3	20	3 starch, 2 high-fat meat
Barbecue	1 slice	390	15	34	6	0	30	650	49	2	17	3 starch, 1 high-fat meat, 2 fat
Deluxe	1 slice	350	14	36	6	0	20	650	43	3	15	3 starch, 1 high-fat meat, 1 fat

(Continued)

✔ = Healthiest Bets

14" FEAST PIZZAS CLASSIC HAND-TOSSED *(Continued)*	Amount	Cal.	Fat (g)	% Cal. Fat	Sat. Fat (g)	Trans Fat (g)	Chol. (mg)	Sod. (mg)	Carb. (g)	Fiber (g)	Pro. (g)	Servings/Exchanges
Extravaganzza	1 slice	420	20	42	8	0	40	930	45	3	20	3 starch, 2 high-fat meat, 1 fat
Hawaiian	1 slice	350	12	30	5	0	25	700	45	3	16	3 starch, 1 high-fat meat, 1 fat
Meatzza	1 slice	430	21	43	9	0	40	960	44	3	20	3 starch, 2 high-fat meat, 1 fat
Pepperoni	1 slice	400	19	42	8	0	35	880	43	3	18	3 starch, 1 high-fat meat, 2 fat
Philly Cheese	1 slice	350	13	33	7	0	30	620	40	2	17	3 starch, 1 high-fat meat, 1 fat
Vegi	1 slice	340	12	31	5	0	20	630	44	3	15	3 starch, 1 high-fat meat, 1 fat

14" FEAST PIZZAS CRUNCHY THIN CRUST

America's Favorite	1 slice	280	18	57	7	0	30	660	22	2	12	1 1/2 starch, 1 high-fat meat, 2 fat
Bacon Cheeseburger	1 slice	310	19	55	8	0	40	570	20	2	15	1 1/2 starch, 1 high-fat meat, 2 fat
Barbecue	1 slice	280	15	48	6	0	30	520	27	1	12	2 starch, 1 high-fat meat 1 1/2 fat
Deluxe	1 slice	240	14	52	6	0	20	520	21	2	10	1 1/2 starch, 1 high-fat meat, 1 fat
Extravaganzza	1 slice	310	20	58	8	0	40	800	23	2	15	1 1/2 starch, 1 high-fat meat, 2 fat
Hawaiian	1 slice	240	12	45	5	0	25	570	23	2	11	1 1/2 starch, 1 high-fat meat, 1 fat
Meatzza	1 slice	320	21	59	9	0	40	830	22	2	15	1 1/2 starch, 1 high-fat meat, 2 1/2 fat

✔ = Healthiest Bets

(Continued)

14" FEAST PIZZAS CRUNCHY THIN CRUST *(Continued)*	Amount	Cal.	Fat (g)	% Cal. Fat	Sat. Fat (g)	Trans Fat (g)	Chol. (mg)	Sod. (mg)	Carb. (g)	Fiber (g)	Pro. (g)	Servings/Exchanges
Pepperoni	1 slice	290	19	58	8	0	35	750	21	2	13	1 1/2 starch, 1 high-fat meat, 2 fat
Philly Cheese	1 slice	240	13	48	7	0	30	490	18	1	12	1 starch, 1 high-fat meat, 1 fat
Vegi	1 slice	230	12	46	5	0	20	500	22	2	10	1 1/2 starch, 1 high-fat meat, 1 fat
14" FEAST PIZZAS ULTIMATE DEEP DISH												
America's Favorite	1 slice	400	21	47	7	0	30	990	42	5	15	3 starch, 1 high-fat meat, 2 1/2 fat
Bacon Cheeseburger	1 slice	430	22	46	8	0	40	900	40	5	18	3 starch, 1 high-fat meat, 2 1/2 fat
Barbecue	1 slice	400	18	40	6	0	30	850	47	4	15	3 starch, 1 high-fat meat, 1 1/2 fat

Deluxe	1 slice	360	17	42	6	0	20	850	41	5	13	3 starch, 1 high-fat meat, 2 fat
Extravaganzza	1 slice	430	23	48	8	0	40	1130	43	5	18	3 starch, 1 high-fat meat, 3 fat
Hawaiian	1 slice	360	15	37	5	0	25	900	43	5	14	3 starch, 1 high-fat meat, 1 1/2 fat
Meatzza	1 slice	440	24	49	9	0	40	1160	42	5	18	3 starch, 1 high-fat meat, 3 fat
Pepperoni	1 slice	410	22	48	8	0	35	1080	41	5	16	3 starch, 1 high-fat meat, 2 1/2 fat
Philly Cheese	1 slice	360	16	40	7	0	30	820	38	4	15	3 starch, 1 high-fat meat, 2 1/2 fat
Vegi	1 slice	350	15	38	5	0	20	830	42	5	13	3 starch, 1 high-fat meat, 1 fat

✔ = Healthiest Bets

(Continued)

	Amount	Cal.	Fat (g)	% Cal. Fat	Sat. Fat (g)	Trans Fat (g)	Chol. (mg)	Sod. (mg)	Carb. (g)	Fiber (g)	Pro. (g)	Servings/Exchanges
14" ULTIMATE DEEP DISH												
American Cheese	1 slice	320	14	39	5	0	15	740	40	5	11	2 starch, 1 medium-fat meat, 2 fat
Anchovies	1 slice	320	14	39	5	0	15	775	40	5	11	2 starch, 1 medium-fat meat, 2 fat
Bacon	1 slice	380	18	42	6.5	0	30	910	40	5	17	2 starch, 2 medium-fat meat, 2 fat
Banana Peppers	1 slice	320	14	39	5	0	15	920	40	5	11	2 starch, 1 medium-fat meat, 2 fat
Beef	1 slice	370	18.5	45	7	0	25	840	40	5	14	2 starch, 1 medium-fat meat, 3 fat
Black Olives	1 slice	330	14.5	39	5	0	15	800	41	5	11	2 starch, 1 medium-fat meat, 2 fat

	Serving										Exchanges
Cheddar Cheese	1 slice	320	14	39	5	0	15	740	40	5	11	2 starch, 1 medium-fat meat, 2 fat
Cheese	1 slice	320	14	39	5	0	15	740	40	5	11	2 starch, 1 medium-fat meat, 2 fat
Extra Cheese	1 slice	350	16.5	42	6.5	0	20	860	41	5	13	2 starch, 1 medium-fat meat, 3 fat
Garlic	1 slice	335	14	37	5	0	15	740	40	5	11	2 starch, 1 medium-fat meat, 2 fat
Green Chile Peppers	1 slice	320	14	39	5	0	15	740	40	5	11	2 starch, 1 medium-fat meat, 2 fat
Green Olives	1 slice	340	16	42	5	0	15	865	41	5	11	2 starch, 1 medium-fat meat, 2 fat
Green Pepper	1 slice	320	14	39	5	0	15	741	40	5	11	2 starch, 1 medium-fat meat, 2 fat
Green Pepper, Onion & Mushroom	1 slice	320	14	39	5	0	15	741	43	5	11	2 starch, 1 medium-fat meat, 2 fat

(*Continued*)

✔ = Healthiest Bets

14" ULTIMATE DEEP DISH *(Continued)*	Amount	Cal.	Fat (g)	% Cal. Fat	Sat. Fat (g)	Trans Fat (g)	Chol. (mg)	Sod. (mg)	Carb. (g)	Fiber (g)	Pro. (g)	Servings/Exchanges
Grilled Chicken	1 slice	345	14.5	37	5	0	30	870	40	5	16	3 starch, 2 medium-fat meat, 2 fat
Ham	1 slice	335	14.5	38	5	0	15	880	40	5	13	2 starch, 1 medium-fat meat, 2 fat
✓Ham & Pineapple	1 slice	350	14.5	37	5	0	15	880	43	5	13	3 starch, 1 medium-fat meat, 2 fat
Jalapeño Peppers	1 slice	320	14	39	5	0	15	875	40	5	11	2 starch, 1 medium-fat meat, 2 fat
Mushrooms	1 slice	320	14	39	5	0	15	740	41	5	11	2 starch, 1 medium-fat meat, 2 fat
✓Onions	1 slice	320	14	39	5	0	15	740	41	5	11	2 starch, 1 medium-fat meat, 2 fat
Pepperoni	1 slice	370	18.5	45	6.5	0	25	930	40	5	13	2 starch, 1 medium-fat meat, 3 fat

Philly Steak	1 slice	335	14.5	38	5	0	20	825	40	5	13	2 starch, 1 medium-fat meat, 2 fat
Pineapple	1 slice	335	14	37	5	0	15	740	43	5	11	2 starch, 1 medium-fat meat, 2 fat
Provolone Cheese	1 slice	320	14	39	5	0	15	740	40	5	11	2 starch, 1 medium-fat meat, 2 fat
Sausage	1 slice	380	19.5	46	7	0	25	930	42	6	13	2 starch, 1 medium-fat meat, 3 fat
Sausage & Pepperoni	1 slice	430	24	50	8.5	0	35	1120	42	6	15	3 starch, 1 medium-fat meat, 3 fat
Tomatoes	1 slice	320	14	39	5	0	15	740	40	5	11	2 starch, 1 medium-fat meat, 2 fat

SALADS

Blue Cheese Dressing	1 serving	230	24	93	5	0	30	450	2	0	2	5 fat
Buttermilk Ranch Dressing	1 serving	220	24	98	4	0	10	420	2	0	1	5 fat

✓ = Healthiest Bets

(Continued)

SALADS (Continued)	Amount	Cal.	Fat (g)	% Cal. Fat	Sat. Fat (g)	Trans Fat (g)	Chol. (mg)	Sod. (mg)	Carb. (g)	Fiber (g)	Pro. (g)	Servings/Exchanges
Creamy Caesar Dressing	1 serving	210	22	94	3.5	0	10	510	2	0	1	4 1/2 fat
✓Garden Fresh Salad	1	70	4	51	2	0	10	85	6	1	6	1 veg, 1 medium-fat meat
Golden Italian Dressing	1 serving	220	23	94	3.5	0	0	370	2	0	0	4 1/2 fat
✓Grilled Chicken Caesar	1	105	4	34	2	0	25	320	6	1	12	1 veg, 2 lean meat
✓Light Italian Dressing	1 serving	20	1	45	0	0	0	780	2	0	0	1/2 fat
SIDE DISHES												
Barbeque Buffalo Wings	1 serving	88	4.5	46	1.5	0	50	0	2	0	9	1 medium-fat meat
Blue Cheese Dipping Sauce	1 serving	230	24	93	5	0	30	450	2	0	2	5 fat
✓Breadsticks	1	130	7	48	1.5	0	0	90	14	1	3	1 starch, 1 fat
✓Cheesy Bread	1	140	7	45	2.3	0	5	140	14	1	4	1 starch, 1 1/2 fat

✓Cinna Stix	1	140	7	45	1.5	0	0	80	17	1	3	1 starch, 1 1/2 fat
Garlic Dipping Sauce	3 T	440	50	100	10	7	0	390	0	0	0	10 fat
Hot Buffalo Wings	1 serving	85	4.5	47	1.5	0	50	250	2	0	9	1 medium-fat meat
Hot Dipping Sauce	1 serving	120	12	90	2	0	0	790	3	0	0	2 1/2 fat
✓Marinara Dipping Sauce	3 T	25	0	0	0	0	0	260	5	0	1	1 veg
✓Pizza Chicken Kickers	1 serving	45	2	40	0	0	10	160	3	0	4	1 lean meat
Ranch Dipping Sauce	1 serving	200	21	94	3	0	10	420	2	0	1	4 fat
Sweet Icing	4 T	250	3	10	2.5	0	0	0	57	0	0	4 carb

✓ = Healthiest Bets

Dunkin' Donuts

www.dunkindonuts.com

Light & Lean Choice

1 English Muffin with Egg and Cheese
Orange Juice (4 oz)

Calories 335	Cholesterol (mg) 140
Fat (g) 9	Sodium (mg) 1,012
% calories from fat ...24	Carbohydrate (g).........47
Saturated fat (g) 4.5	Fiber (g).....................0
Trans fat (g) 0	Protein (g) 17

Exchanges: 2 starch, 1 fruit, 2 lean meat

Healthy & Hearty Choice

1 Raisin Bran Muffin
Low-Fat Milk (8 oz)

Calories 582	Cholesterol (mg) 72
Fat (g) 17	Sodium (mg) 587
% calories from fat ...26	Carbohydrate (g).........91
Saturated fat (g) 2	Fiber (g).....................5
Trans fat (g) 0	Protein (g) 16

Exchanges: 5 starch, 1 low-fat milk

(Continued)

Dunkin' Donut

BAGELS

	Amount	Cal.	Fat (g)	% Cal. Fat	Sat. Fat (g)	Trans Fat (g)	Chol. (mg)	Sod. (mg)	Carb. (g)	Fiber (g)	Pro. (g)	Servings/Exchanges
✓ Blueberry	1	330	3	8	0.5	0	0	600	66	2	10	4 starch
✓ Cinnamon Raisin	1	330	3	8	0.5	0	0	430	65	3	10	4 starch
✓ Everything	1	370	6	14	0.5	0	0	650	67	3	14	4 1/2 starch
✓ Harvest	1	350	6	15	1	0	0	500	61	7	13	4 1/2 starch
✓ Multigrain	1	380	6	14	1	0	0	650	68	5	14	4 1/2 starch
✓ Onion	1	320	4	11	0.5	0	0	610	61	3	12	4 starch
✓ Plain	1	320	3	8	0.5	0	0	650	62	2	12	4 starch
✓ Poppyseed	1	370	7	17	0.5	0	0	650	65	3	14	4 1/2 starch, 1 fat
Reduced Carb w/ Cheese	1	380	12	28	4.5	0	20	780	45	14	25	3 starch, 2 lean meat, 1 fat

✔Salsa	1	310	3	8	0.5	0	0	790	60	2	13	4 starch
Salt	1	320	3	8	0.5	0	0	4520	62	2	12	4 starch
✔Sesame	1	380	8	18	0.5	0	0	650	64	3	14	4 starch, 1 1/2 fat
✔Wheat	1	330	4	10	1	0	0	610	62	4	12	4 starch

BREAKFAST SANDWICHES

Bacon Egg Cheese Bagel	1	540	18	30	7	0	200	1400	69	2	18	4 1/2 starch, 2 high-fat meat
Bacon Egg Cheese Croissant	1	520	33	57	10	7	205	940	40	0	16	2 1/2 starch, 1 high-fat meat, 5 fat
Bacon Egg Cheese English Muffin	1	360	16	40	6	0	200	1300	36	0	17	2 starch, 2 high fat meat
Biscuit	1	250	13	46	3.5	8	0	780	29	1	5	2 starch, 2 1/2 fat
Egg Cheese Bagel	1	470	15	28	6	0	190	1120	65	2	20	4 starch, 1 medium-fat meat, 2 fat

(Continued)

✔ = Healthiest Bets

148 *Dunkin' Donuts*

BREAKFAST SANDWICHES *(Continued)*	Amount	Cal.	Fat (g)	% Cal. Fat	Sat. Fat (g)	Trans Fat (g)	Chol. (mg)	Sod. (mg)	Carb. (g)	Fiber (g)	Pro. (g)	Servings/Exchanges
Egg Cheese Biscuit	1	410	25	54	9	7	190	1250	32	1	14	2 starch, 1 medium-fat meat, 4 fat
Egg Cheese Croissant	1	550	34	55	11	7	320	950	41	0	20	3 starch, 2 medium-fat meat, 4 1/2 fat
✔Egg Cheese English Muffin	1	280	9	28	4.5	0	140	1010	34	1	15	2 starch, 1 medium-fat meat, 1 fat
Ham Egg Cheese Bagel	1	510	16	28	6	0	200	1390	65	2	26	4 starch, 2 medium-fat meat, 1 fat
Ham Egg Cheese Croissant	1	520	32	55	10	7	215	1010	40	0	20	2 1/2 starch, 2 medium-fat meat, 4 fat
Ham Egg Cheese English Muffin	1	310	10	29	5	0	160	1270	34	1	21	2 starch, 2 medium-fat meat
Plain Croissant	1	330	18	49	4.8	7	5	270	37	0	5	2 starch, 3 1/2 fat

	Amount	Cal.	Fat (g)	% Cal. Fat	Sat. Fat (g)	Trans Fat (g)	Chol. (mg)	Sod. (mg)	Carb. (g)	Fiber (g)	Prot. (g)	Servings/Exchanges
Sausage Egg Cheese Bagel	1	660	35	47	13	0.5	225	1450	63	3	28	4 starch, 2 high-fat meat, 3 1/2 fat
Sausage Egg Cheese Biscuit	1	610	43	63	14	7	235	1760	32	1	23	2 starch, 2 high-fat meat, 5 1/2 fat
Sausage Egg Cheese Croissant	1	690	51	66	17	7	230	1080	40	0	22	2 1/2 starch, 3 high-fat meat, 4 fat
Sausage Egg Cheese English Muffin	1	530	32	54	12	0.5	235	1610	37	1	23	2 1/2 starch, 3 high-fat meat, 1 fat
Steak, Cheddar & Egg	1	600	40	60	13	7	245	980	41	0	24	3 starch, 2 medium-fat meat, 5 fat
Supreme Omelet on Croissant	1	590	38	57	13	6	260	1040	42	1	21	3 starch, 2 medium-fat meat, 5 fat

CAKE DONUTS

	Amount	Cal.	Fat (g)	% Cal. Fat	Sat. Fat (g)	Trans Fat (g)	Chol. (mg)	Sod. (mg)	Carb. (g)	Fiber (g)	Prot. (g)	Servings/Exchanges
Apple Crumb	1	290	15	46	13	0.5	15	320	41	1	3	3 carb, 2 fat
Blueberry	1	290	16	49	3.5	2.5	10	400	35	1	3	2 carb, 3 fat

✔ = Healthiest Bets

(*Continued*)

CAKE DONUTS *(Continued)*	Amount	Cal.	Fat (g)	% Cal. Fat	Sat. Fat (g)	Trans Fat (g)	Chol. (mg)	Sod. (mg)	Carb. (g)	Fiber (g)	Pro. (g)	Servings/Exchanges
Chocolate Coconut	1	300	19	57	6	5	0	370	31	1	4	2 carb, 3 fat
Chocolate Frosted	1	360	20	50	5	5	25	350	40	1	4	3 carb, 3 1/2 fat
Chocolate Glazed	1	290	16	49	3.5	4	0	370	33	1	3	3 carb, 2 1/2 fat
Cinnamon	1	330	20	54	5	4	25	340	34	1	4	2 carb, 4 fat
Double Chocolate	1	310	17	49	3.5	5	0	370	37	2	3	2 carb, 3 fat
Frosted Lemon	1	240	14	52	3.5	2.5	0	150	28	0	2	2 carb, 2 fat
Glazed	1	350	19	48	5	4	25	340	41	1	4	3 carb, 3 fat
✔ Glazed Ginger Bread	1	260	11	38	2.5	4	20	320	35	1	3	2 carb, 2 fat
Glazed Lemon	1	240	14	52	3.5	2.5	0	150	28	0	2	2 carb, 2 1/2 fat
Old Fashioned	1	300	19	57	5	4	25	330	28	1	4	2 carb, 3 fat
Powdered	1	330	19	51	5	4	25	330	36	1	4	3 carb, 2 1/2 fat

Whole Wheat Glazed	1	310	19	55	4	4	0	380	32	2	4	2 carb, 3 1/2 fat

COOKIES

✔Chocolate Chunk	2	220	11	45	7	0	35	105	28	1	3	2 carb, 2 fat
✔Chocolate Chunk w/ Walnuts	2	230	12	46	6	0	35	110	27	1	3	2 carb, 2 fat
✔Oatmeal Raisin Pecan	2	220	10	40	5	0	30	110	29	1	3	2 carb, 2 fat
✔White Chocolate Chunk	2	230	12	46	7	0	35	120	28	1	3	2 carb, 2 fat

COOLATTA

Coffee w/ 2% milk	16 oz	190	2	9	1.5	0	10	80	41	0	4	2 1/2 carb
Coffee w/ cream	16 oz	350	22	56	14	0	75	65	40	0	3	2 1/2 carb, 4 fat
Coffee w/ milk	16 oz	210	4	17	2.5	0	15	80	42	0	4	3 carb
Coffee w/ skim milk	16 oz	170	0	0	0	0	0	80	41	0	4	3 carb
Lemonade	16 oz	240	0	0	0	0	0	35	59	0	0	4 carb
Strawberry Fruit	16 oz	290	0	0	0	0	0	30	72	1	0	4 1/2 carb

✔ = Healthiest Bets

(Continued)

COOLATTA *(Continued)*	Amount	Cal.	Fat (g)	% Cal. Fat	Sat. Fat (g)	Trans Fat (g)	Chol. (mg)	Sod. (mg)	Carb. (g)	Fiber (g)	Pro. (g)	Servings/Exchanges
Tropicana Orange	16 oz	370	0	0	0	0	0	50	92	3	1	6 carb
Vanilla Bean	16 oz	440	17	34	15	1	0	95	70	1	1	4 1/2 carb, 3 fat
CREAM CHEESE												
✔Chive	4 T	170	17	90	11	0	45	230	4	2	4	3 fat
✔Garden Vegetable	4 T	170	15	79	11	0	45	340	4	0	2	3 1/2 fat
✔Lite	4 T	110	9	73	7	0	30	230	6	0	4	2 fat
✔Plain	4 T	190	17	80	13	0	55	190	4	0	4	3 1/2 fat
✔Salmon	4 T	170	17	90	11	0	45	180	2	0	4	3 1/2 fat
✔Shedd's Buttermatch Blend	1 T	80	9	100	2	6	0	100	0	0	0	2 fat
✔Strawberry	4 T	190	17	80	9	0	45	150	9	0	4	3 1/2 fat
DANISH												
Apple	1	330	20	54	9	0	30	260	32	1	4	2 carb, 4 fat

Cheese	1	340	22	58	10	0	35	270	30	1	4	2 carb, 4 fat
Strawberry Cheese	1	320	20	56	9	0	30	260	31	1	4	2 carb, 4 fat

FANCIES

Apple Fritter	1	300	14	42	3	2.5	0	360	41	1	4	2 1/2 carb, 2 1/2 fat
Bow Tie Donut	1	300	17	51	3.5	5	0	340	34	1	4	2 carb, 3 fat
Chocolate Frosted Roll	1	290	15	46	3	0.5	0	340	36	1	4	2 carb, 3 fat
Chocolate Iced Bismark	1	340	15	39	3.5	1.5	0	290	50	1	3	3 carb, 3 fat
Coffee Roll	1	270	14	46	3	0	0	340	33	1	4	2 carb, 2 1/2 fat
Éclair	1	270	11	36	2.5	0.5	0	290	39	1	3	2 1/2 carb, 2 fat
Glazed Fritter	1	260	14	48	3	2.5	0	330	31	1	4	2 carb, 2 1/2 fat
Maple Frosted Coffee Roll	1	290	14	43	3	0	0	340	36	1	4	2 carb, 3 fat
Vanilla Frosted Coffee Roll	1	290	14	43	3	0	0	340	36	1	4	2 carb, 3 fat

(Continued)

✔ = Healthiest Bets

	Amount	Cal.	Fat (g)	% Cal. Fat	Sat. Fat (g)	Trans Fat (g)	Chol. (mg)	Sod. (mg)	Carb. (g)	Fiber (g)	Pro. (g)	Servings/Exchanges
FLAVORED COFFEE												
All flavors	10 oz	20	0	0	0	0	0	65	4	0	1	1/2 carb
HOT ESPRESSO DRINKS												
✓ Cappuccino	10 oz	80	5	56	2.5	0	20	70	7	0	4	1 milk
✓ Cappuccino w/ Soy Milk	10 oz	70	3	38	0	0	0	80	6	1	4	1 milk
Cappuccino w/ Soy Milk & Sugar	10 oz	120	3	22	0	0	0	80	20	1	4	1/2 carb, 1 milk
Cappuccino w/ Sugar	10 oz	130	5	34	2.5	0	15	65	21	0	4	1/2 carb, 1 milk, 1 fat
Caramel Crème Hot Latte	10 oz	260	9	31	6	0	20	125	40	0	8	1 1/2 carb, 1 milk, 1 fat
Caramel Swirl Latte	10 oz	230	6	23	3.5	0	25	140	36	0	8	2 carb, 1 milk
Caramel Swirl Latte w/ Soy Milk	10 oz	210	4	17	0	0	0	160	34	1	8	1 1/2 carb, 1 milk

✔ Espresso	2 oz	0	0	0	0	0	5	1	0	0	free
Espresso w/ Sugar	2 oz	30	0	0	0	0	5	7	0	0	1/2 carb
✔ Hot Latte Lite	10 oz	70	0	0	0	0	80	10	0	6	1 milk
✔ Latte	10 oz	120	6	45	3.5	25	95	10	0	6	1 milk , 1/2 fat
✔ Latte w/ Soy Milk	10 oz	90	4	40	0	0	110	8	1	6	1 milk
Latte w/ Soy Milk & Sugar	10 oz	150	4	24	0	0	110	22	1	6	1/2 carb, 1 milk
Latte w/ Sugar	10 oz	160	6	33	3.5	25	95	22	0	6	1 carb, 1/2 milk, 1 fat
Mocha Almond Hot Latte	10 oz	290	10	31	7	50	115	46	1	8	2 carb, 1 milk, 1 1/2 fat
Mocha Swirl Latte	10 oz	230	7	27	4	25	110	37	1	6	2 carb, 1/2 milk, 1 fat
Mocha Swirl Latte w/ Soy Milk	10 oz	210	5	21	1	0	130	35	2	7	2 carb, 1/2 milk, 1 fat
ICED ESPRESSO DRINKS											
Caramel Crème Iced Latte	16 oz	260	9	31	6	20	125	40	0	8	2 1/2 carb, 1/2 milk, 1 fat

(Continued)

✔ = Healthiest Bets

ICED ESPRESSO DRINKS (Continued)	Amount	Cal.	Fat (g)	% Cal. Fat	Sat. Fat (g)	Trans Fat (g)	Chol. (mg)	Sod. (mg)	Carb. (g)	Fiber (g)	Pro. (g)	Servings/Exchanges
Iced Caramel Swirl Latte	16 oz	240	7	26	4	0	25	150	37	0	8	2 carb, 1/2 milk, 1 fat
Iced Caramel Swirl Latte w/ Skim Milk	16 oz	180	0	0	0	0	0	150	36	0	8	2 carb, 1/2 milk
✓Iced Latte	16 oz	120	7	52	4	0	25	105	11	0	6	1/2 carb, 1 milk
✓Iced Latte Lite	16 oz	80	0	0	0	0	0	110	13	0	10	1 milk
✓Iced Latte w/ Skim Milk	16 oz	70	0	0	0	0	0	110	11	0	8	1 milk
Iced Latte w/ Skim Milk & Sugar	16 oz	120	0	0	0	0	0	110	23	0	8	1 carb, 1 milk
Iced Latte w/ Sugar	16 oz	170	7	37	4	0	25	110	23	0	6	1 carb, 1 milk
Iced Mocha Swirl Latte	16 oz	240	8	30	4.5	0	25	125	38	1	7	1 1/2 carb, 1 milk, 1 fat
Iced Mocha Swirl Latte w/ Skim Milk	16 oz	180	1	5	1	0	0	115	37	1	7	1 carb, 1 milk
Mocha Almond Iced Latte	16 oz	290	10	31	7	0	20	115	46	1	8	2 carb, 1 milk, 1 1/2 fat
✓Turbo Ice	16 oz	120	7	52	3.5	0	20	25	14	0	1	1 carb, 1 1/2 fat

MUFFIN

Banana Walnut	1	540	25	41	3.5	0	65	520	69	3	10	4 1/2 carb, 4 fat
Blueberry	1	470	17	32	3	0	60	500	73	2	8	5 carb, 2 fat
Chocolate Chip	1	630	26	37	8	0	70	560	89	2	10	5 1/2 carb, 4 fat
Coffee Cake	1	580	19	29	3	0	65	520	78	1	9	5 carb, 4 fat
Corn	1	510	18	31	3.5	0	75	860	75	1	8	5 carb, 2 1/2 fat
Cranberry Orange	1	440	17	34	3	0	65	480	66	3	8	4 carb, 3 fat
✔ English Muffin	1	160	1.5	8	0	0	0	340	31	2	6	2 carb
Honey Bran Raisin	1	480	15	28	2.5	0	60	480	79	5	8	5 carb, 2 fat
Reduced Fat Blueberry	1	440	5	10	2	0	60	490	78	3	8	5 carb, 1 fat

MUNCHKINS

Cinnamon Cake	4	270	15	50	3.5	4	25	210	31	1	3	2 carb, 2 1/2 fat
✔ Glazed	5	200	9	40	2	2.5	0	220	27	1	3	2 carb, 1 1/2 fat

(Continued)

✔ = Healthiest Bets

MUNCHKINS *(Continued)*	Amount	Cal.	Fat (g)	% Cal. Fat	Sat. Fat (g)	Trans Fat (g)	Chol. (mg)	Sod. (mg)	Carb. (g)	Fiber (g)	Pro. (g)	Servings/Exchanges
Glazed Cake	3	280	13	41	3	4	20	190	38	1	3	2 1/2 carb, 2 fat
✔ Glazed Chocolate Cake	3	200	10	45	2	5	0	250	26	1	3	1 1/2 carb, 2 fat
✔ Jelly Filled	5	210	9	38	2	2.5	0	240	30	1	3	2 carb, 1 1/2 fat
✔ Lemon Filled	4	170	8	42	1.5	2.5	0	190	23	0	2	1 1/2 carb, 1 fat
Plain Cake	4	270	16	53	4	4	25	240	27	1	3	1 1/2 carb, 3 fat
Powdered Cake	4	270	14	46	3.5	4	25	210	31	1	3	2 carb, 2 1/2 fat
Sugar Raised	7	220	12	49	2.5	0.5	0	290	26	1	4	1 1/2 carb, 2 1/2 fat
OTHER HOT BEVERAGES												
Dunkaccuino	10 oz	230	10	39	3	5	5	210	35	0	2	2 carb, 1 1/2 fat
Hot Chocolate	10 oz	220	8	32	2	4	0	280	38	2	2	2 1/2 carb, 1 1/2 fat
✔ Regular Tea w/ milk	10 oz	25	1	36	0.5	0	5	15	2	0	1	1/2 carb
Regular Tea w/ milk & sugar	10 oz	70	1	12	0.5	0	5	15	14	0	1	1 carb

	Amount	Cal	Fat (g)	% Fat	Sat Fat (g)	Trans Fat (g)	Chol (mg)	Sod (mg)	Carb (g)	Fiber (g)	Pro (g)	Exchanges/Choices
✔ Regular Tea w/ skim milk	10 oz	25	0	0	0	0	0	70	4	0	2	1/2 carb
Regular Tea w/ sugar	10 oz	50	0	0	0	0	0	0	13	0	0	1 carb
Vanilla Chai	10 oz	230	8	31	6	0	5	50	40	0	1	2 1/2 carb, 1 1/2 fat
PANINIS												
Meatball	1	480	19	35	9	0	40	1180	56	3	22	3 1/2 starch, 2 medium-fat meat, 1 1/2 fat
✔ Southwest Chicken	1	420	10	21	5	0	45	970	57	3	23	3 1/2 starch, 2 medium-fat meat
Steak	1	450	12	24	5	0.5	45	1630	56	3	30	3 1/2 starch, 3 lean meat
STICKS												
Cinnamon Cake	1	450	30	60	7	5	35	310	42	1	4	3 carb, 5 fat
Glazed Cake	1	490	29	53	7	5	35	310	51	1	4	3 1/2 carb, 5 fat
Glazed Chocolate	1	470	29	55	7	5	0	490	49	2	4	3 carb, 5 fat

✔ = Healthiest Bets

(*Continued*)

STICKS *(Continued)*	Amount	Cal.	Fat (g)	% Cal. Fat	Sat. Fat (g)	Trans Fat (g)	Chol. (mg)	Sod. (mg)	Carb. (g)	Fiber (g)	Pro. (g)	Servings/Exchanges
Jelly	1	530	29	49	7	5	35	320	61	1	4	4 carb, 5 fat
Plain Cake	1	420	29	62	7	5	35	310	35	1	4	2 carb, 6 fat
Powdered Cake	1	450	29	58	7	5	35	310	42	1	4	3 carb, 5 fat
YEAST DONUTS												
✔ Apple N' Spice	1	200	8	36	1.5	2.5	0	270	29	1	3	2 carb, 1 fat
✔ Bavarian Kreme	1	210	9	38	2	2.5	0	270	30	1	3	2 carb, 1 fat
✔ Black Raspberry	1	210	8	34	1.5	4	0	280	32	1	3	2 carb, 1 fat
Blueberry Crumb	1	240	10	37	3	0.5	0	260	36	1	3	2 carb, 2 fat
Boston Kreme	1	240	9	33	2	3.5	0	280	36	1	3	2 carb, 2 fat
✔ Chocolate Frosted	1	200	9	40	2	5	0	260	29	1	3	2 carb, 1 fat
Chocolate Kreme Filled	1	270	13	43	3	4	0	260	35	1	3	2 carb, 2 1/2 fat
✔ French Cruller	1	150	8	48	2	3	20	105	17	1	2	1 carb, 2 fat

✔Glazed	1	180	8	40	1.5	4	0	250	25	1	3	1 1/2 carb, 1 1/2 fat
Jelly Filled	1	210	8	34	1.5	4	0	280	32	1	3	2 carb, 2 fat
Lemon Burst	1	300	14	42	5	2.5	0	300	35	3	3	2 carb, 3 fat
✔Maple Frosted	1	210	9	38	2	2.5	0	260	30	1	3	2 carb, 2 fat
✔Marble Frosted	1	200	9	40	2	2.5	0	260	29	1	3	2 carb, 2 fat
✔Strawberry Frosted	1	210	9	38	2	2.5	0	260	30	1	3	2 carb, 2 fat
✔Sugar Raised	1	170	8	42	1.5	0.5	0	250	22	1	3	1 1/2 carb, 1 1/2 fat
Vanilla Kreme Filled	1	270	13	43	3	3.5	0	250	36	1	3	2 carb, 2 fat

✔ = Healthiest Bets

KFC

www.KFC.com

Light & Lean Choice

**2 Oven-Roasted Drumsticks
1 Corn on the Cob (large)
Green Beans (1 order)**

Calories	480	Cholesterol (mg)	155
Fat (g)	21	Sodium (mg)	1,460
% calories from fat	40	Carbohydrate (g)	41
Saturated fat (g)	4	Fiber (g)	9
Trans fat (g)	0	Protein (g)	38

Exchanges: 2 1/2 starch, 1 vegetable, 4 lean meat,
1 1/2 fat

Healthy & Hearty Choice

**1 Oven-Roasted Chicken Breast
Baked Beans (1/2 order)
Cole Slaw (1 order)**

Calories	685	Cholesterol (mg)	150
Fat (g)	30	Sodium (mg)	1,810
% calories from fat	39	Carbohydrate (g)	56
Saturated fat (g)	8.5	Fiber (g)	7
Trans fat (g)	3	Protein (g)	45

Exchanges: 4 1/2 starch, 5 lean meat, 3 fat

(*Continued*)

KFC

	Amount	Cal.	Fat (g)	% Cal. Fat	Sat. Fat (g)	Trans Fat (g)	Chol. (mg)	Sod. (mg)	Carb. (g)	Fiber (g)	Pro. (g)	Servings/Exchanges
BREAD												
Biscuit	1	190	10	47	2	1.5	1.5	580	23	0	2	1 1/2 starch, 2 fat
CHICKEN												
Boneless Fiery Buffalo Wings (6)	1 order	520	25	43	4.5	3.5	35	2520	44	1	30	3 starch, 3 high-fat meat
Boneless Sweet & Spicy Wings (6)	1 order	540	24	40	4.5	4.5	65	1850	50	1	30	3 1/2 starch, 3 medium-fat meat, 1 1/2 fat
Boneless Wings in HBBQ Sauce (7)	1 order	510	24	42	4.5	4.5	65	1670	42	1	30	3 starch, 3 medium-fat meat, 1 1/2 fat
Chicken Pot Pie	1	770	40	46	15	14	115	1680	70	5	33	4 1/2 starch, 3 medium-fat meat, 3 1/2 fat

Item	Serving											Exchanges
Crispy Strips (2)	1 order	270	16	53	3.5	3	50	850	11	0	19	1 starch, 2 medium-fat meat, 1 fat
Crispy Strips (3)	1 order	400	24	54	5	4.5	75	1250	17	0	29	1 starch, 4 medium-fat meat, 1/2 fat
Extra Crispy Breast	1	460	28	54	8	4.5	135	1230	19	0	34	1 starch, 4 medium-fat meat, 1 1/2 fat
✔ Extra Crispy Drumstick	1	160	10	56	2.5	1.5	70	420	5	0	12	2 medium-fat meat
Extra Crispy Thigh	1	370	26	63	7	3	120	710	12	0	21	1 starch, 3 medium-fat meat, 2 fat
Extra Crispy Whole Wing	1	190	12	56	4	2	55	390	10	0	10	1/2 starch, 1 medium-fat meat, 1 1/2 fat
Family Popcorn	1	1210	68	50	16	14	200	3870	73	1	77	5 starch, 9 medium-fat meat, 3 1/2 fat
Fiery Buffalo Wings (6)	1 order	440	26	53	7	3.5	155	1800	26	3	27	1 1/2 starch, 3 medium-fat meat, 3 fat

(Continued)

✔ = Healthiest Bets

CHICKEN *(Continued)*	Amount	Cal.	Fat (g)	% Cal. Fat	Sat. Fat (g)	Trans Fat (g)	Chol. (mg)	Sod. (mg)	Carb. (g)	Fiber (g)	Pro. (g)	Servings/Exchanges
Hot Wings (6)	1	450	29	58	6	4	145	1120	23	1	24	1 1/2 starch, 3 medium-fat meat, 2 fat
Individual Popcorn	1	380	21	49	5	4.5	60	1200	23	0	24	1 1/2 starch, 3 medium-fat meat, 1 fat
✔Kids Popcorn	1	240	14	52	3	3	40	770	15	0	15	1 starch, 2 medium-fat meat, 1/2 fat
Large Popcorn	1	560	31	49	7	7	90	1790	34	1	36	2 starch, 4 medium-fat meat, 2 1/2 fat
Oven Roasted Breast	1	380	19	45	6	2.5	145	1150	11	0	40	1 starch, 5 lean meat, 1/2 fat
✔Oven Roasted Breast w/out skin or breading	1	140	3	19	1	0	95	410	0	0	29	4 very-lean meat
✔Oven Roasted Drumstick	1	140	8	51	2	1	75	40	4	0	14	2 medium-fat meat

	Amt	Cal	Fat	%Fat	Sat	Trans	Chol	Sod	Carb	Fib	Pro	Exchanges/Choices
Oven Roasted Thigh	1	360	25	62	1.5		165	1060	12	0	22	1 starch, 3 medium-fat meat, 2 fat
Oven Roasted Whole Wing	1	150	9	54	2.5	1	60	370	5	0	11	2 medium-fat meat
Sweet & Spicy Wings (6)	1 order	460	26	50	7	3.5	155	950	32	3	27	2 starch, 3 medium-fat meat, 2 fat
Wings in HBBQ Sauce (6)	1 order	540	33	55	7	4.5	150	1130	36	1	25	2 starch, 3 medium-fat meat, 3 fat

DESSERTS

	Amt	Cal	Fat	%Fat	Sat	Trans	Chol	Sod	Carb	Fib	Pro	Exchanges/Choices
Apple Minis	1 order	400	22	49	5	7	0	250	46	2	3	3 carb, 4 fat
Apple Pie Slice	1	290	11	34	3	2.5	0	230	44	2	2	3 carb, 1 1/2 fat
Double Chocolate Chip Cake	1	400	29	65	5	0.5	45	230	31	2	4	2 carb, 5 1/2 fat
Lemon Meringue Pie	1	240	9	33	2.5	1.5	0	230	40	1	1	2 1/2 carb, 1 1/2 fat
Lil' Bucket Chocolate Cream	1	270	13	43	8	0.5	0	180	37	2	2	2 1/2 starch, 2 fat
Lil' Bucket Fudge Brownie	1	270	9	30	4	0.5	30	170	44	1	2	3 carb, 2 fat

(Continued)

✔ = Healthiest Bets

DESSERTS (Continued)	Amount	Cal.	Fat (g)	% Cal. Fat	Sat. Fat (g)	Trans Fat (g)	Chol. (mg)	Sod. (mg)	Carb. (g)	Fiber (g)	Pro. (g)	Servings/Exchanges
Lil' Bucket Lemon Crème	1	400	14	31	7	1.5	5	210	65	2	4	4 carb, 3 fat
Lil' Bucket Strawberry Short Cake	1	200	6	27	4	0	20	110	34	0	2	2 carb, 1 fat
Pecan Pie Slice	1	480	21	39	4.5	1	40	360	68	2	5	4 1/2 carb, 3 1/2 fat
✔Quaker Chew S'mores Granola Bar	1	110	2	16	0.5	0	0	70	22	1	1	1 1/2 carb
Sweet Potato Pie	1	340	16	42	4	3	5	210	44	5	1	3 carb, 3 fat
SALADS & MORE												
✔Caesar Side Salad w/out Dressing & Croutons	1	50	3	54	2	0	10	135	2	1	4	1 lean meat
Crispy BLT Salad w/out Dressing	1	350	17	43	1.5	3	60	1170	21	4	27	1 starch, 1 veg, 3 medium-fat meat

Item	Amount	Cal	Fat	%Fat			Chol	Sod	Carb	Fiber	Pro	Exchanges/Choices
Crispy Caesar Salad w/out Dressing	1	370	19	46	7	3.5	65	1110	20	3	29	1 starch, 1 veg, 4 medium-fat meat
✔Hidden Valley Fat Free Ranch Dressing	1 serving	35	0	0	0	0	0	410	8	0	1	1/2 carb
Hidden Valley Golden Italian Light Dressing	1 serving	45	2.5	50	0	0	0	660	6	0	0	1/2 carb, 1/2 fat
Hidden Valley Original Ranch Dressing	1 serving	200	20	90	3	3	25	470	3	0	1	4 fat
✔House Side Salad w/out Dressing	1	15	0	0	0	0	0	0	5	2	1	1 veg
KFC Creamy Parmesan Caesar Dressing	1 serving	260	26	90	5	0.5	15	530	5	0	2	1/2 carb, 5 fat
✔KFC Parmesan Garlic Croutons	1 packet	70	3	38	0	0	0	160	9	0	1	1/2 starch, 1 fat

(Continued)

✔ = Healthiest Bets

SALADS & MORE *(Continued)*	Amount	Cal.	Fat (g)	% Cal. Fat	Sat. Fat (g)	Trans Fat (g)	Chol. (mg)	Sod. (mg)	Carb. (g)	Fiber (g)	Pro. (g)	Servings/Exchanges
Mashed Potatoes with Gravy	1	690	31	40	9	4.5	55	2110	77	6	27	5 starch, 2 high-fat meat, 2 1/2 fat
Mashed Potatoes with Honey BBQ	1	710	29	36	8	4.5	55	2010	88	6	26	6 starch, 1 high-fat meat, 5 fat
Rice with Gravy	1	770	25	29	8	4	55	2750	107	8	30	7 starch, 1 high-fat meat, 4 fat
✔ Roasted BLT Salad w/out Dressing	1	210	7	30	2.5	0	70	900	8	4	28	2 veg, 4 very lean meat, 1/2 fat
✔ Roasted Caesar Salad w/out Dressing & Croutons	1	220	9	36	4.5	0.5	75	850	6	3	29	1 veg, 4 very lean meat, 1 fat
Tender Roast Filet Meal	1	360	7	17	2	0.5	85	2010	41	4	33	3 starch, 3 very lean meat

SANDWICHES

Crispy Twister	1	670	38	51	7	4	60	1650	55	3	21	3 1/2 starch, 2 high-fat meat, 4 1/2 fat
Double Crunch	1	530	28	47	6	3	55	1240	42	3	27	3 starch, 3 high-fat meat, 1/2 fat
✔Honey BBQ	1	300	6	18	1.5	0.5	50	640	41	4	21	3 starch, 2 lean meat
✔Honey BBQ Snacker	1	220	3.5	14	1	0	35	490	32	2	15	2 starch, 1 lean meat
✔KFC Snacker	1	320	16	45	3	1.5	25	700	31	2	14	2 starch, 1 high fat meat, 1 1/2 fat
Oven Roasted Twister	1	510	23	40	4	0	70	1400	46	4	29	3 starch, 3 medium-fat meat, 1 1/2 fat
✔Tender Roast	1	390	19	43	4	0.5	70	810	24	1	31	1 1/2 starch, 4 lean meat, 1 1/2 fat
✔Tender Roast w/out sauce	1	260	5	17	1.5	0.5	65	690	23	1	31	1 1/2 starch, 4 very-lean meat

(Continued)

✔ = Healthiest Bets

SANDWICHES *(Continued)*	Amount	Cal.	Fat (g)	% Cal. Fat	Sat. Fat (g)	Trans Fat (g)	Chol. (mg)	Sod. (mg)	Carb. (g)	Fiber (g)	Pro. (g)	Servings/Exchanges
Triple Crunch	1	650	34	47	7	4.5	75	1640	49	3	36	3 starch, 4 medium-fat meat, 2 1/2 fat
SIDE DISHES												
✔Baked Beans	1	230	1	3	1	0	0	720	46	7	8	3 starch
✔Baked Cheetos	1	120	4.5	33	1	0	0	210	17	0	2	1 starch, 1 fat
Cole Slaw	1	190	11	52	2	0	5	300	22	3	1	1 starch, 2 veg, 2 fat
✔Corn on the Cob 3"	1	70	2	25	0.5	0	0	5	13	3	2	1 starch
✔Corn on the Cob 5.5"	1	150	3	18	1	0	0	10	26	7	5	2 starch
✔Green Beans	1	50	2	36	0	0	5	570	7	2	2	1 veg, 1/2 fat
Macaroni and Cheese	1	400	18	40	5	2.5	15	1920	45	4	15	3 starch, 1 high-fat meat, 2 fat
✔Mashed Potatoes w/ Gravy	1	120	5	37	1	0.5	0	380	18	1	2	1 starch, 1 fat

✔ Mashed Potatoes w/out Gravy	1	110	4	32	1	0.5	0	260	16	1	2	1 starch, 1 fat
Potato Salad	1	180	9	45	1.5	0	5	470	22	1	2	1 1/2 starch, 2 fat
Potato Wedges (small)	1	240	12	45	3	4	0	830	30	3	1	2 starch, 2 fat
✔ Seasoned Rice	1	150	1	6	0	0	0	640	32	2	4	2 starch

✔ = Healthiest Bets

McDonald's

www.mcdonalds.com

**1 California Cobb Salad with Grilled Chicken
Newman's Own Cobb Dressing
(2 T or 1/2 packet)
1 Fruit 'n Yogurt Parfait without Granola**

Calories	470	Cholesterol (mg)	165
Fat (g)	17	Sodium (mg)	1,615
% calories from fat	33	Carbohydrate (g)	46
Saturated fat (g)	7	Fiber (g)	4
Trans fat (g)	0	Protein (g)	40

Exchanges: 2 carb, 2 vegetable, 4 lean meat, 1 fat

**1 Hamburger (regular)
French Fries (1/2 medium order)
1 Side Salad
Low-Fat Balsamic Vinaigrette (2 T or 1/2 packet)**

Calories	750	Cholesterol (mg)	60
Fat (g)	28	Sodium (mg)	1,545
% calories from fat	34	Carbohydrate (g)	96
Saturated fat (g)	7	Fiber (g)	5
Trans fat (g)	4	Protein (g)	29

Exchanges: 4 starch, 1 vegetable, 1 medium-fat meat, 3 fat

(Continued)

McDonald's

	Amount	Cal.	Fat (g)	% Cal. Fat	Sat. Fat (g)	Trans Fat (g)	Chol. (mg)	Sod. (mg)	Carb. (g)	Fiber (g)	Pro. (g)	Servings/Exchanges
BREAKFAST												
Bacon, Egg & Cheese Biscuit	1	440	24	49	8	5	245	1250	36	1	19	2 starch, 3 high-fat meat
Bacon, Egg & Cheese McGriddles	1	450	21	42	7	1.5	245	1260	46	1	20	3 starch, 2 high-fat meat, 1/2 fat
Big Breakfast	1	730	46	56	14	7	465	1470	53	3	27	3 1/2 starch, 2 high-fat meat, 6 fat
Biscuit	1	240	11	41	2.5	5	0	680	31	1	4	2 starch, 2 fat
Deluxe Breakfast	1	1220	61	45	17	11	480	1920	136	4	33	9 starch, 2 high-fat meat, 7 fat
Deluxe Warm Cinnamon Roll	1	590	24	36	7	6	55	660	86	4	9	5 1/2 starch, 4 fat

✔ Egg McMuffin	1	300	12	36	5	0	230	840	30	2	17	2 starch, 2 medium-fat meat
✔ English Muffin	1	170	4.5	23	1	0	0	290	27	2	5	2 starch
✔ Grape Jam	0.5 oz	35	0	0	0	0	0	0	9	0	0	1/2 carb
✔ Hash Browns	1 order	140	8	51	1.5	2	0	290	15	2	1	1 starch, 1 1/2 fat
Hotcakes (margarine and syrup)	1 order	600	17	25	4	4	20	620	102	2	9	5 starch, 2 carb, 3 fat
Hotcakes and Sausage	1 order	770	33	38	9	4	50	930	104	0	15	7 starch, 2 high-fat meat, 3 fat
Sausage Biscuit	1	410	26	57	8	5	30	990	34	1	10	2 starch, 1 high-fat meat, 4 fat
Sausage Biscuit w/ Egg	1	500	31	55	10	5	250	1080	36	1	18	2 starch, 2 high-fat meat, 3 fat
✔ Sausage Burrito	1	300	16	48	6	1	175	760	26	2	13	1 1/2 starch, 1 high-fat meat, 1 1/2 fat

✔ = Healthiest Bets

(Continued)

BREAKFAST *(Continued)*	Amount	Cal.	Fat (g)	% Cal. Fat	Sat. Fat (g)	Trans Fat (g)	Chol. (mg)	Sod. (mg)	Carb. (g)	Fiber (g)	Pro. (g)	Servings/Exchanges
Sausage McGriddles	1	420	22	47	7	1.5	30	990	44	1	11	3 starch, 1 high-fat meat, 3 fat
Sausage McMuffin	1	380	22	52	8	0.5	45	800	31	2	14	2 starch, 1 high-fat meat, 3 fat
Sausage McMuffin w/ Egg	1	450	27	54	10	0.5	255	950	31	2	20	2 starch, 2 high-fat meat, 2 fat
Sausage Patty	1 order	170	15	79	6	0	30	310	0	0	7	1 high-fat meat, 1 1/2 fat
Sausage, Egg & Cheese McGriddles	1	560	32	51	11	1.5	260	1300	47	1	21	3 starch, 3 high-fat meat, 1 fat
✔ Scrambled Eggs	2	160	12	67	4	0	435	200	5	0	15	2 medium-fat meat
✔ Strawberry Preserves	0.5 oz	35	0	0	0	0	0	0	9	0	0	1/2 carb
Warm Cinnamon Roll	1	420	18	38	4.5	4.5	60	400	57	2	8	4 starch, 3 fat

CHICKEN McNUGGETS/SELECTS

	Amount	Cal	Fat (g)	% Fat Cal	Sat Fat (g)	Trans Fat (g)	Chol (mg)	Sod (mg)	Carb (g)	Fiber (g)	Pro (g)	Exchanges/Choices
Chicken McNuggets (10 piece)	1 order	420	24	51	5	2.5	60	1120	26	0	25	1 1/2 starch, 3 medium-fat meat, 2 fat
Chicken McNuggets (20 piece)	1 order	840	49	52	11	5	125	2240	51	0	50	3 1/2 starch, 6 medium-fat meat, 3 1/2 fat
Chicken McNuggets (4 piece)	1 order	170	10	52	2	1	25	450	10	0	10	1/2 starch, 1 medium-fat meat, 1 fat
Chicken McNuggets (6 piece)	1 order	250	15	54	3	1.5	35	670	15	0	15	1 starch, 2 medium-fat meat, 1 fat
Chicken Selects Premium Breast Strips	3 pc	380	20	47	3.5	2.5	55	930	28	0	23	2 starch, 2 medium-fat meat, 2 fat
Chicken Selects Premium Breast Strips	5 pc	630	33	47	6	4.5	90	1550	46	0	39	3 starch, 3 medium-fat meat, 3 fat
Chicken Selects Premium Breast Strips	10 pc	1270	66	46	12	9	180	3100	92	0	77	6 starch, 8 medium-fat meat, 5 fat

(Continued)

✔ = Healthiest Bets

CHICKEN SAUCES

	Amount	Cal.	Fat (g)	% Cal. Fat	Sat. Fat (g)	Trans Fat (g)	Chol. (mg)	Sod. (mg)	Carb. (g)	Fiber (g)	Pro. (g)	Servings/Exchanges
Barbeque	2 T	45	0	0	0	0	0	250	10	0	0	1/2 starch
Creamy Ranch Sauce	2 T	200	21	94	0	0	10	300	3	0	0	4 fat
Honey	1 T	45	0	0	0	0	0	0	12	0	0	1 carb
✔Honey Mustard	2 T	50	5	90	0.5	0	10	95	3	0	0	1 fat
✔Hot Mustard	2 T	40	4	90	0	0	5	240	7	0	0	1/2 carb, 1/2 fat
✔Light Mayonnaise	1 pkg	45	5	100	0.5	0	10	100	0	0	0	1 fat
✔Southwestern Chipotle Barbeque	2 T	70	0	0	0	0	0	260	16	1	0	1 carb
✔Spicy Buffalo Sauce	2 T	60	6	90	1	0	0	910	1	1	0	1 fat
✔Sweet 'N Sour	2 T	50	0	0	0	0	0	140	11	0	0	1/2 carb
✔Tangy Honey Mustard	2 T	70	2	25	0	0	0	160	13	1	1	1 carb

DESSERTS / SHAKES

DESSERTS / SHAKES	Amount											Exchanges
✔ Apple Dippers	1 pkg	35	0	0	0	0	0	0	8	0	0	1/2 carb
✔ Apple Dippers w/ low fat Caramel Dip	3.2 oz	100	0.5	4	0	0	5	40	24	0	0	1 1/2 starch
Baked Apple Pie	1	250	11	39	3	4.5	0	150	34	2	2	1 starch, 1 fruit, 2 1/2 fat
✔ Chocolate Chip Cookie	1	160	7	39	2	1.5	10	95	22	1	2	1 1/2 carb, 2 fat
Chocolate Triple Thick Shake 16 oz		580	14	21	8	1	50	250	104		13	6 carb, 3 fat
Chocolate Triple Thick Shake 21 oz		770	18	21	11	1	70	330	134		18	8 carb, 3 1/2 fat
Chocolate Triple Thick Shake 32 oz		1160	27	20	16	2	100	510	203		27	12 1/2 carb, 5 1/2 fat
Chocolate Triple Thick Shake 12 oz		440	10	20	6	0.5	40	190	76		10	4 1/2 carb, 2 fat
✔ Fruit 'n Yogurt Parfait	5.3 oz	160	2	11	1	0	5	85	31	0	4	2 carb
✔ Fruit 'n Yogurt Parfait w/out granola	5.0 oz	130	2	13	1	0	5	55	25	0	4	1 1/2 carb

✔ = Healthiest Bets

(Continued)

DESSERTS/SHAKES *(Continued)*	Amount	Cal.	Fat (g)	% Cal. Fat	Sat. Fat (g)	Trans Fat (g)	Chol. (mg)	Sod. (mg)	Carb. (g)	Fiber (g)	Pro. (g)	Servings/Exchanges
Hot Caramel Sundae	6.4 oz	340	7	18	4.5	0	30	140	62	0	7	4 carb, 1 1/2 fat
Hot Fudge Sundae	6.3 oz	330	9	24	6	0	25	170	55	1	8	3 1/2 carb, 1 1/2 fat
✔Kiddie Cone	1.0 oz	45	1	20	0.5	0	5	20	8	0	1	1/2 carb
Low Fat Caramel Dip	2 T	70	0.5	6	0	0	5	40	15	0	0	1 carb
M&M McFlurry	12.3 oz	620	20	29	12	1	55	190	96	1	14	6 carb, 4 fat
McDonaldland Chocolate Chip Cookies	2 oz	270	11	36	6	0	35	170	39	1	3	2 1/2 carb, 2 fat
McDonaldland Cookies	2 oz	250	8	28	2	2.5	0	270	42	1	4	3 carb, 1 fat
✔Oatmeal Raisin Cookie	1	140	5	32	1	1	10	125	22	1	2	1 1/2 carb, 1 fat
Oreo McFlurry	11.9 oz	560	16	25	9	2	50	250	88	0	14	5 1/2 carb, 3 fat
✔Peanuts for Sundaes	0.3 oz	45	3.5	70	0.5	0	0	0	2	0	1	1/2 fat
Strawberry Sundae	6.3 oz	280	6	19	3.5	0	25	85	51	0	6	3 1/2 carb, 1/2 fat

Item												
Strawberry Triple Thick Shake	32 oz	1110	26	21	16	2	100	350	194	2	25	13 carb, 3 fat
Strawberry Triple Thick Shake	21 oz	740	18	21	11	1	70	230	128	1	17	8 1/2 carb, 2 fat
Strawberry Triple Thick Shake	16 oz	560	13	20	8	1	50	170	97	0	13	6 1/2 carb, 2 fat
Strawberry Triple Thick Shake	12 oz	420	10	21	6	0.5	40	130	73	0	10	5 carb, 1 1/2 fat
✔ Vanilla Reduced Fat Ice Cream Cone	3.2 oz	150	3.5	21	2	0	15	60	24	0	4	1 1/2 carb, 1 fat
Vanilla Triple Thick Shake	21 oz	740	18	21	11	1	70	230	128	0	17	8 1/2 carb, 2 fat
Vanilla Triple Thick Shake	32 oz	1110	26	21	16	2	100	370	193	0	25	13 carb, 3 1/2 fat
Vanilla Triple Thick Shake	16 oz	550	13	21	8	1	50	190	96	0	13	6 1/2 carb, 1 1/2 fat
Vanilla Triple Thick Shake	12 oz	420	10	21	6	0.5	40	140	72	0	9	4 1/2 carb, 2 fat

✔ = Healthiest Bets

(*Continued*)

	Amount	Cal.	Fat (g)	% Cal. Fat	Sat. Fat (g)	Trans Fat (g)	Chol. (mg)	Sod. (mg)	Carb. (g)	Fiber (g)	Pro. (g)	Servings/Exchanges
FRENCH FRIES												
Large French Fries	1 order	570	25	39	5	6	0	330	70	7	6	4 1/2 starch, 5 fat
Medium French Fries	1 order	380	16	37	2	4	0	220	47	5	4	3 starch, 3 fat
✔Small French Fries	1 order	250	11	39	2	2.5	0	140	30	3	2	2 starch, 2 fat
SALAD DRESSING												
Newman's Own Cobb Dressing	4 T	120	9	67	1.5	0	10	440	9	0	1	1/2 carb, 2 fat
Newman's Own Creamy Caesar Dressing	2 oz	190	18	85	3.5	0	20	500	4	0	2	4 fat
✔Newman's Own Low Fat Balsamic Vinaigrette	3 T	40	3	67	0	0	0	730	4	0	0	1/2 fat
✔Newman's Own Low Fat Italian	1.5 oz	50	2.5	45	0.5	0	1	680	7	0	1	1/2 starch, 1/2 fat

Newman's Own Ranch Dressing	2 oz	170	15	79	2.5	0	6	530	9	0	1	1/2 starch, 3 fat
SALADS												
Bacon Ranch w/ Crispy Chicken	1	340	16	42	5	1.5	70	1140	23	3	28	1 veg, 3 medium-fat meat
✔Bacon Ranch w/ Grilled Chicken	1	260	9	31	4	0	90	1000	12	3	33	1/2 starch, 1 veg, 4 lean meat
✔Bacon Ranch w/out Chicken	1	140	7	45	3.5	0	25	290	10	3	9	2 veg, 1 high-fat meat
✔Butter Garlic Croutons	0.5 oz	60	1	15	0	0	0	160	10	1	2	1 starch
Caesar w/ Crispy Chicken	1	300	13	39	4	1.5	55	1020	22	3	25	1 starch, 1 veg, 3 lean meat, 1 fat
✔Caesar w/ Grilled Chicken	1	220	6	24	3	0	75	800	12	3	30	2 veg, 3 lean meat
✔Caesar w/out Chicken	1	90	4	40	2.5	0	10	180	7	3	7	1 veg, 1 medium-fat meat
California Cobb w/ Crispy Chicken	1	360	18	45	6	1.5	130	1250	22	4	30	1 starch, 1 veg, 3 medium-fat meat, 1/2 fat

(Continued)

✔ = Healthiest Bets

SALADS *(Continued)*	Amount	Cal.	Fat (g)	% Cal. Fat	Sat. Fat (g)	Trans Fat (g)	Chol. (mg)	Sod. (mg)	Carb. (g)	Fiber (g)	Pro. (g)	Servings/Exchanges
California Cobb w/ Grilled Chicken	1	280	11	35	5	0	150	1120	12	4	35	1/2 starch, 1 veg, 4 lean meat
✓California Cobb w/out Chicken	1	160	9	50	4	0	85	410	9	4	11	2 veg, 2 lean meat
✓Fruit & Walnut	1	310	13	37	2	0	5	85	44	6	5	3 fruit, 1 high-fat meat, 1 fat
✓Side Salad	1	20	0	0	0	0	0	10	4	1	1	1 veg
SANDWICHES												
Big Mac	1	560	30	48	10	1.5	80	1010	47	3	25	3 1/2 starch, 2 medium-fat meat, 4 fat
Big N' Tasty	1	470	23	44	8	1.5	80	790	41	3	24	3 starch, 3 medium-fat meat, 1 fat

Big N' Tasty w/ Cheese	1	520	26	45	10	1.5	95	1010	42	3	27	2 1/2 starch, 3 medium-fat meat, 2 fat
✔Cheeseburger	1	310	12	34	6	1	40	740	35	1	15	2 starch, 1 medium-fat meat, 1 1/2 fat
Double Cheeseburger	1	460	23	45	11	1.5	80	1140	37	1	25	2 1/2 starch, 2 medium-fat meat 2 1/2 fat
Double Quarter Pounder w/ Cheese	1	770	40	46	19	3	160	1330	46	3	47	3 starch, 5 medium-fat meat, 3 1/2 fat
✔Fillet-O-Fish	1	400	18	40	4	1	40	640	42	1	14	3 starch, 1 medium-fat meat, 2 fat
✔Hamburger	1	260	9	31	3.5	0.5	30	530	33	1	13	2 starch, 2 medium-fat meat, 1/2 fat
✔McChicken	1	370	16	38	3.5	1	50	810	41	3	15	3 starch, 1 medium-fat meat 1 1/2 fat

✔ = Healthiest Bets

(Continued)

SANDWICHES *(Continued)*	Amount	Cal.	Fat (g)	% Cal. Fat	Sat. Fat (g)	Trans Fat (g)	Chol. (mg)	Sod. (mg)	Carb. (g)	Fiber (g)	Pro. (g)	Servings/Exchanges
Premium Grilled Chicken Classic	1	420	9	19	2	0	80	1240	52	3	32	3 1/2 starch, 3 lean meat
Premium Grilled Chicken Club	1	590	22	33	8	0	120	1690	54	3	45	3 1/2 starch, 5 lean meat, 1 fat
Premium Grilled Chicken Ranch BLT	1	490	13	23	4	0	90	1610	54	3	39	3 1/2 starch, 4 lean meat
Premium Grilled Crispy Chicken Classic	1	500	16	28	3	1.5	60	1380	62	3	27	4 starch, 2 medium-fat meat, 1 fat
Premium Grilled Crispy Chicken Club	1	680	29	38	9	1.5	100	1830	64	3	40	4 starch, 4 medium-fat meat, 2 fat
Premium Grilled Crispy Chicken Ranch BLT	1	580	20	31	5	1.5	70	1750	64	3	34	4 starch, 3 medium-fat meat, 1 fat
Premium Spicy Chicken	1	510	17	30	3	1.5	55	1430	59	3	25	4 starch, 2 medium-fat meat, 1 fat

✓Quarter Pounder	1	420	18	7	1	70	730	40	3	24	2 1/2 starch, 2 medium-fat meat, 1 1/2 fat
Quarter Pounder w/ Cheese	1	510	25	44	12	1.5	95	1150	43	3	29	3 starch, 3 medium-fat meat, 2 fat

✓ = Healthiest Bets

Papa John's Pizza

www.papajohns.com

Light & Lean Choice

12" Original Crust Garden Fresh Pizza (3 slices)

Calories	600	Cholesterol (mg)	30
Fat (g)	21	Sodium (mg)	1,350
% calories from fat	32	Carbohydrate (g)	84
Saturated fat (g)	6	Fiber (g)	6
Trans fat (g)	0	Protein (g)	24

Exchanges: 5 starch, 2 vegetable, 1 medium-fat meat, 3 fat

Healthy & Hearty Choice

14" Original Crust Garden Fresh Pizza (3 slices)

Calories	840	Cholesterol (mg)	45
Fat (g)	27	Sodium (mg)	2,040
% calories from fat	30	Carbohydrate (g)	120
Saturated fat (g)	8	Fiber (g)	6
Trans fat (g)	0	Protein (g)	33

Exchanges: 7 starch, 2 vegetable, 1 medium-fat meat, 4 fat

(Continued)

Papa John's Pizza

12" ORIGINAL CRUST PIZZA

	Amount	Cal.	Fat (g)	% Cal. Fat	Sat. Fat (g)	Trans Fat (g)	Chol. (mg)	Sod. (mg)	Carb. (g)	Fiber (g)	Pro. (g)	Servings/Exchanges
BBQ Chicken & Bacon	1 slice	240	8	30	2.5	0	20	690	32	1	11	2 starch, 1 high-fat meat
Cheese	1 slice	210	8	34	2.5	0	15	520	27	1	9	1 1/2 starch, 1 medium-fat meat, 1/2 fat
✓Garden Fresh	1 slice	200	7	31	2	0	10	500	28	2	8	2 starch, 1 fat
✓Grilled Chicken Alfredo	1 slice	210	8	34	3	0	20	510	26	1	11	1 1/2 starch, 1 medium-fat meat, 1/2 fat
Grilled Chicken Club	1 slice	230	8	31	2.5	0	20	590	28	1	11	2 starch, 1 lean meat, 1/2 fat
Hawaiian BBQ Chicken	1 slice	240	8	30	2.5	0	20	690	33	1	11	2 starch, 1 medium-fat meat, 1/2 fat

Pepperoni	1 slice	220	9	36	3	0	15	580	27	1	9	1 1/2 starch, 1 high-fat meat
Sausage	1 slice	240	11	41	3.5	0	15	590	27	2	9	1 1/2 starch, 1 high-fat meat, 1 fat
Spicy Italian	1 slice	260	8	27	7	0	20	690	27	3	11	1 1/2 starch, 1 high-fat meat, 1 fat
✔ Spinach Alfredo	1 slice	210	8	34	3	0	15	450	26	1	8	1 1/2 starch, 1 medium-fat meat
✔ Spinach Alfredo Chicken Tomato	1 slice	220	8	32	3.5	0	20	490	27	2	10	1 1/2 starch, 1 medium-fat meat, 1/2 fat
The Meats w/ Beef	1 slice	250	11	39	3.5	0	25	670	27	2	11	1 1/2 starch, 2 medium-fat meat, 1 fat
The Meats w/out Beef	1 slice	240	11	41	3.5	0	20	650	27	2	11	1 1/2 starch, 1 medium-fat meat, 1 fat
The Works	1 slice	230	8	31	3.5	0	15	620	28	2	10	2 starch, 1 high-fat meat

✔ = Healthiest Bets

(Continued)

14" ORIGINAL CRUST PIZZA

	Amount	Cal.	Fat (g)	% Cal. Fat	Sat. Fat (g)	Trans Fat (g)	Chol. (mg)	Sod. (mg)	Carb. (g)	Fiber (g)	Pro. (g)	Servings/Exchanges
BBQ Chicken & Bacon	1 slice	340	11	29	3.5	0	30	960	44	2	15	3 starch, 1 high-fat meat, 1/2 fat
Cheese	1 slice	310	12	34	3.5	0	20	770	39	2	13	2 1/2 starch, 1 high-fat meat, 1/2 fat
Garden Fresh	1 slice	280	9	28	2.5	0	15	680	40	2	11	3 starch, 1 high-fat meat
Grilled Chicken Alfredo	1 slice	300	11	33	4	0	30	700	36	2	15	2 starch, 1 medium-fat meat, 1 1/2 fat
Grilled Chicken Club	1 slice	320	12	33	3.5	0	30	840	40	2	16	3 starch, 1 medium-fat meat, 1 1/2 fat
Hawaiian BBQ Chicken	1 slice	340	11	29	3.5	0	30	960	46	2	16	3 starch, 1 medium-fat meat, 1 1/2 fat

Pepperoni	1 slice	320	13	36	4	0	20	820	38	2	13	2 1/2 starch, 1 high-fat meat, 1 fat
Sausage	1 slice	330	15	40	4.5	0	20	820	38	3	13	2 1/2 starch, 1 high-fat meat, 1 fat
Spicy Italian	1 slice	370	11	26	10	0	30	970	39	4	15	2 1/2 starch, 1 high-fat meat, 1 1/2 fat
Spinach Alfredo	1 slice	290	11	34	4.5	0	20	630	36	2	11	2 starch, 1 high-fat meat, 1 fat
Spinach Alfredo Chicken Tomato	1 slice	300	11	33	4.5	0	25	680	37	2	13	2 1/2 starch, 1 medium-fat meat, 1 fat
The Meats w/ Beef	1 slice	370	17	41	6	0	35	980	38	3	17	2 1/2 starch, 2 high-fat meat
The Meats w/out Beef	1 slice	350	16	41	5	0	30	940	38	2	15	2 1/2 starch, 1 high-fat meat, 1 1/2 fat
The Works	1 slice	330	11	30	6	0	25	900	40	3	14	3 starch, 2 medium-fat meat

(Continued)

✔ = Healthiest Bets

14" PAN CRUST PIZZA

	Amount	Cal.	Fat (g)	% Cal. Fat	Sat. Fat (g)	Trans Fat (g)	Chol. (mg)	Sod. (mg)	Carb. (g)	Fiber (g)	Pro. (g)	Servings/Exchanges
BBQ Chicken & Bacon	1 slice	420	19	40	6	2	30	1200	44	1	17	3 starch, 1 high-fat meat, 2 fat
Cheese	1 slice	390	19	43	6	2	20	990	39	1	15	2 1/2 starch, 1 high-fat meat, 2 fat
Garden Fresh	1 slice	360	17	42	5	2	15	920	40	2	13	2 1/2 starch, 1 high-fat meat, 1 1/2 fat
Grilled Chicken Alfredo	1 slice	380	19	45	6	2	30	940	36	1	16	2 starch, 1 medium-fat meat, 2 1/2 fat
Grilled Chicken Club	1 slice	410	20	43	6	2	30	1060	39	2	17	2 1/2 starch, 1 medium-fat meat, 3 fat
Hawaiian BBQ Chicken	1 slice	420	19	40	6	2	30	1130	44	1	17	3 starch, 1 medium-fat meat, 2 1/2 fat

Pepperoni	1 slice	400	21	47	7	2	20	1060	38	1	15	2 1/2 starch, 1 high-fat meat, 2 1/2 fat
Sausage	1 slice	410	23	50	7	2	20	1040	38	2	14	2 1/2 starch, 1 high-fat meat, 3 fat
Spicy Italian	1 slice	460	19	37	13	2	30	1200	39	3	16	2 1/2 starch, 2 high-fat meat, 1/2 fat
Spinach Alfredo	1 slice	370	19	46	7	2	20	870	26	1	13	1 1/2 starch, 2 medium-fat meat, 1 fat
Spinach Alfredo Chicken Tomato	1 slice	390	20	46	7	2	25	920	37	2	14	2 1/2 starch, 2 medium-fat meat, 1 fat
The Meats w/ Beef	1 slice	450	25	50	8	2	35	1210	38	2	18	2 1/2 starch, 2 high-fat meat, 1 1/2 fat
The Works	1 slice	410	19	41	8	2	25	1120	39	2	15	2 1/2 starch, 1 high-fat meat, 2 fat

(Continued)

✔ = Healthiest Bets

14" THIN CRUST PIZZA

	Amount	Cal.	Fat (g)	% Cal. Fat	Sat. Fat (g)	Trans Fat (g)	Chol. (mg)	Sod. (mg)	Carb. (g)	Fiber (g)	Pro. (g)	Servings/Exchanges
BBQ Chicken & Bacon	1 slice	290	14	43	3.5	0	30	740	29	0	12	2 starch, 1 medium-fat meat, 2 fat
Cheese	1 slice	260	14	48	3.5	0	20	550	24	1	11	1 1/2 starch, 1 high-fat meat, 1 fat
Garden Fresh	1 slice	230	12	46	3	0	15	480	25	2	9	1 1/2 starch, 1 medium-fat meat, 1 fat
Grilled Chicken Alfredo	1 slice	250	13	46	4	0	30	480	21	1	12	1 1/2 starch, 1 medium-fat meat, 1 1/2 fat
Grilled Chicken Club	1 slice	270	14	46	3.5	0	30	620	25	1	13	1 1/2 starch, 1 medium-fat meat, 1 1/2 fat
Hawaiian BBQ Chicken	1 slice	290	14	43	3.5	0	30	740	31	1	13	2 starch, 1 medium-fat meat, 1 1/2 fat

Pepperoni	1 slice	270	15	50	4.5	0	20	600	23	1	10	1 1/2 starch, 1 high-fat meat, 1 1/2 fat
Sausage	1 slice	280	18	57	5	0	30	600	23	2	10	1 1/2 starch, 1 high-fat meat, 2 fat
Spicy Italian	1 slice	320	14	39	11	0	30	750	24	3	12	1 1/2 starch, 1 high-fat meat, 1 1/2 fat
Spinach Alfredo	1 slice	240	14	52	4.5	0	20	410	21	1	9	1 1/2 starch, 1 high-fat meat, 1 fat
Spinach Alfredo Chicken Tomato	1 slice	250	14	50	4.5	0	25	460	22	1	11	1 1/2 starch, 1 high-fat meat, 1 fat
The Meats w/ Beef	1 slice	320	20	56	6	0	35	760	23	2	14	1 1/2 starch, 1 high-fat meat, 2 1/2 fat
The Meats w/out Beef	1 slice	300	18	54	5	0	30	720	23	2	13	1 1/2 starch, 1 high-fat meat, 2 fat
The Works	1 slice	280	14	45	6	0	25	680	25	3	12	1 1/2 starch, 1 high-fat meat, 1 1/2 fat

✔ = Healthiest Bets

(Continued)

SIDE ITEMS

	Amount	Cal.	Fat (g)	% Cal. Fat	Sat. Fat (g)	Trans Fat (g)	Chol. (mg)	Sod. (mg)	Carb. (g)	Fiber (g)	Pro. (g)	Servings/Exchanges
Apple Twist Sweetreat	1/2 pie	360	13	32	3	1.5	0	550	54	1	6	3 1/2 carb, 2 fat
✔BBQ Dipping Sauce	2 T	40	0	0	0	0	0	240	11	0	0	1/2 starch
Blue Cheese Dipping Sauce	2 T	170	18	95	3.5	n/a	20	240	1	0	1	3 1/2 fat
✔Breadsticks	1 stick	140	2	12	0	n/a	0	260	26	1	4	1 1/2 starch
✔Buffalo Dipping Sauce	2 T	15	1	60	0.5	n/a	0	890	2	0	0	free
✔Cheese Dipping Sauce	2 T	70	6	77	1.5	0	0	150	1	0	1	1 1/2 fat
Cheesesticks	2 sticks	360	16	40	4.5	0	25	830	42	2	15	3 starch, 1 high-fat meat, 1 fat
✔Cinna Swirl Sweetreat	1/2 pie	400	18	40	4	1.5	0	590	53	1	7	3 1/2 carb, 2 1/2 fat
Garlic Dipping Sauce	2 T	150	17	100	3	n/a	n/a	310	n/a	0	0	3 fat
✔Garlic Parmesan Breadsticks	1	170	6	31	1	n/a	0	370	26	1	5	1 1/2 starch, 1 fat

Item	Serving	Cal	Fat (g)	% Fat Cal	Sat Fat (g)	Trans Fat (g)	Chol (mg)	Sod (mg)	Carb (g)	Fiber (g)	Prot (g)	Exchanges/Choices
Honey Mustard Dipping Sauce	2 T	150	15	90	2	n/a	10	120	5	0	0	3 fat
Papa's Chicken Strips	2 strips	160	8	45	2	n/a	25	350	10	0	10	1/2 starch, 1 medium-fat meat, 1 fat
Papa's Cinnapple	2 slices	200	8	36	1.5	n/a	n/a	320	29	0	3	1 carb, 1 fruit , 1 1/2 fat
Papa's Mild Chipotle Barbecue Wings	2 wings	160	10	56	3	0	85	570	5	0	14	2 medium-fat meat
Papa's Spicy Buffalo Wings	2 wings	160	11	61	3.5	0	90	680	1	0	14	2 medium-fat meat
✔ Pizza Dipping Sauce	2 T	20	0	0	0	n/a	0	140	3	0	0	free
Ranch Dipping Sauce	2 T	110	11	90	2	n/a	10	250	1	0	1	2 fat
Very Berry Sweetreat	1/2 pie	410	12	26	3	2	0	580	67	2	7	4 1/2 carb, 2 fat

✔ = Healthiest Bets n/a = not available

Pizza Hut

www.pizzahut.com

Light & Lean Choice

12" Thin 'N Crispy Chicken Supreme Pizza (3 slices)

Calories......................600	Cholesterol (mg) 75
Fat (g) 21	Sodium (mg) 1,560
% calories from fat ...32	Carbohydrate (g).........66
Saturated fat (g) 11	Fiber (g)......................3
Trans fat (g)...............2	Protein (g) 36

Exchanges: 4 starch, 1 vegetable, 3 medium-fat meat, 1 fat

Healthy & Hearty Choice

12" Fit 'N Delicious Pizza with Ham, Pineapple, and Red Tomato (4 slices)

Calories......................640	Cholesterol (mg) 60
Fat (g) 16	Sodium (mg) 1,880
% calories from fat ...23	Carbohydrate (g).........96
Saturated fat (g) 8	Fiber (g)......................8
Trans fat (g)...............1	Protein (g) 32

Exchanges: 3 1/2 starch, 2 vegetable, 3 lean meat, 1 fat

(*Continued*)

Pizza Hut

12" MEDIUM HAND-TOSSED STYLE PIZZA

	Amount	Cal.	Fat (g)	% Cal. Fat	Sat. Fat (g)	Trans Fat (g)	Chol. (mg)	Sod. (mg)	Carb. (g)	Fiber (g)	Pro. (g)	Servings/Exchanges
✔ Cheese Only	1 slice	240	8	30	4.5	0	25	520	30	2	12	2 starch, 1 medium-fat meat, 1/2 fat
✔ Chicken Supreme	1 slice	230	6	23	3	0	25	550	30	2	14	2 starch, 1 medium-fat meat
Meat Lover's	1 slice	300	13	39	6	0.5	35	760	29	2	15	2 starch, 1 high-fat meat, 1 fat
Pepperoni	1 slice	250	9	32	4.5	0	25	570	29	2	12	2 starch, 1 high-fat meat
Pepperoni Lover's	1 slice	300	13	39	7	0.5	40	710	30	2	15	2 starch, 1 high-fat meat, 1 fat

	Serving	Cal						Sod			Exchanges
Quartered Ham	1 slice	220	6	24	3	0	20	550	29	2 12	2 starch, 1 lean meat, 1/2 fat
Sausage Lover's	1 slice	280	12	38	5	0	30	650	30	2 13	2 starch, 1 high-fat meat, 1/2 fat
Super Supreme	1 slice	300	13	39	6	0	35	780	31	2 15	2 starch, 1 high-fat meat, 1 fat
Supreme	1 slice	270	11	36	5	0.5	25	660	30	2 13	2 starch, 1 high-fat meat, 1/2 fat
✔Veggie Lover's	1 slice	220	6	24	3	0	15	490	31	2 10	2 starch, 1 medium-fat meat

12" MEDIUM PAN PIZZA

	Serving	Cal						Sod			Exchanges
Cheese Only	1 slice	280	13	41	5	0.5	25	500	29	1 11	2 starch, 1 high-fat meat, 1/2 fat
Chicken Supreme	1 slice	280	12	38	4	0	25	530	30	2 13	2 starch, 1 medium-fat meat, 1 1/2 fat

(Continued)

✔ = Healthiest Bets

12" MEDIUM PAN PIZZA *(Continued)*	Amount	Cal.	Fat (g)	% Cal. Fat	Sat. Fat (g)	Trans Fat (g)	Chol. (mg)	Sod. (mg)	Carb. (g)	Fiber (g)	Pro. (g)	Servings/Exchanges
Meat Lover's	1 slice	340	19	50	7	0.5	35	750	29	2	15	2 starch, 1 high-fat meat, 2 fat
Pepperoni	1 slice	290	15	46	5	0.5	25	560	29	2	11	2 starch, 1 high-fat meat, 1 1/2 fat
Pepperoni Lover's	1 slice	340	19	50	7	0.5	40	700	29	2	15	2 starch, 1 high-fat meat, 2 fat
Quartered Ham	1 slice	260	11	38	4	0	20	540	29	1	11	2 starch, 1 medium-fat meat, 1 fat
Sausage Lover's	1 slice	330	17	46	6	0	30	640	29	2	13	2 starch, 1 high-fat meat, 1 1/2 fat
Super Supreme	1 slice	340	18	47	6	0.5	35	760	30	2	14	2 starch, 1 high-fat meat, 2 fat
Supreme	1 slice	320	16	45	6	0.5	25	650	30	2	13	2 starch, 1 high-fat meat, 1 1/2 fat

Veggie Lover's	1 slice	260	12	41	4	0	15	470	30	2	10	2 starch, 1 medium-fat meat, 1 fat

12" MEDIUM THIN 'N CRISPY PIZZA

✓Cheese Only	1 slice	200	8	36	4.5	0.5	25	490	21	1	10	1 1/2 starch, 1 high-fat meat
✓Chicken Supreme	1 slice	200	7	31	3.5	0.5	25	520	22	1	12	1 1/2 starch, 1 medium-fat meat
Meat Lover's	1 slice	270	14	46	6	0.5	35	740	21	2	13	1 1/2 starch, 1 high-fat meat, 1 fat
Pepperoni	1 slice	210	10	42	4.5	0.5	25	550	21	1	10	1 1/2 starch, 1 high-fat meat
Pepperoni Lover's	1 slice	260	14	48	7	0.5	40	690	21	2	13	1 1/2 starch, 1 high-fat meat, 1 fat
Quartered Ham	1 slice	180	6	30	3	0.5	20	530	21	1	9	1 1/2 starch, 1 medium-fat meat

✔ = Healthiest Bets

(Continued)

12" MEDIUM THIN 'N CRISPY PIZZA (Continued)	Amount	Cal.	Fat (g)	% Cal. Fat	Sat. Fat (g)	Trans Fat (g)	Chol. (mg)	Sod. (mg)	Carb. (g)	Fiber (g)	Pro. (g)	Servings/Exchanges
Sausage Lover's	1 slice	240	13	48	6	0	30	630	21	2	11	1 1/2 starch, 1 high-fat meat, 1 fat
Super Supreme	1 slice	260	13	45	6	0.5	35	760	23	2	13	1 1/2 starch, 1 high-fat meat, 1 fat
Supreme	1 slice	240	11	41	5	0.5	25	640	22	2	11	1 1/2 starch, 1 high-fat meat, 1/2 fat
✔Veggie Lover's	1 slice	180	7	35	3	0.5	15	480	23	2	8	1 1/2 starch, 1 medium-fat meat
14" LARGE HAND-TOSSED STYLE PIZZA												
✔Cheese Only	1 slice	220	8	32	4.5	0	25	480	27	1	11	1 1/2 starch, 1 high-fat meat
✔Chicken Supreme	1 slice	210	6	25	3	0	20	500	28	2	13	2 starch, 1 medium-fat meat

	Serving	Cal.	Fat									Exchanges
Meat Lover's	1 slice	280	12	38	6	0.5	35	710	27	2	14	1 1/2 starch, 1 high-fat meat, 1 1/2 fat
Pepperoni	1 slice	230	9	35	4.5	0	25	540	27	2	11	1 1/2 starch, 1 high-fat meat
Pepperoni Lover's	1 slice	280	13	41	6	0.5	35	680	27	2	14	1 1/2 starch, 1 high-fat meat, 1 fat
✔Quartered Ham	1 slice	200	6	27	3	0	20	520	27	1	11	1 1/2 starch, 1 medium-fat meat
Super Supreme	1 slice	270	12	40	5	0	30	720	28	2	14	2 starch, 1 high-fat meat, 1/2 fat
Supreme	1 slice	250	10	36	5	0	25	620	28	2	13	2 starch, 1 high-fat meat
✔Veggie Lover's	1 slice	200	6	27	3	0	15	460	28	2	9	1 1/2 starch, 1 medium-fat meat

(Continued)

✔ = Healthiest Bets

14" LARGE PAN PIZZA

	Amount	Cal.	Fat (g)	% Cal. Fat	Sat. Fat (g)	Trans Fat (g)	Chol. (mg)	Sod. (mg)	Carb. (g)	Fiber (g)	Pro. (g)	Servings/Exchanges
Cheese Only	1 slice	270	13	43	5	0.5	25	470	27	1	11	1 1/2 starch, 1 high-fat meat, 1 fat
Chicken Supreme	1 slice	260	11	38	4	0	20	490	27	1	12	1 1/2 starch, 1 medium-fat meat, 1 fat
Meat Lover's	1 slice	320	18	50	6	0.5	35	690	27	2	14	1 1/2 starch, 2 high-fat meat
Pepperoni	1 slice	280	14	45	5	0	25	530	26	1	11	1 1/2 starch, 1 high-fat meat, 1 fat
Pepperoni Lover's	1 slice	330	18	49	7	0.5	35	670	27	2	14	1 1/2 starch, 1 high-fat meat, 1 1/2 fat
Quartered Ham	1 slice	250	11	39	4	0	20	510	26	1	11	1 1/2 starch, 1 medium-fat meat, 1 fat

	Serving Size	Cal.	Fat (g)	% Cal. Fat	Sat. Fat (g)	Trans Fat (g)	Chol. (mg)	Sod. (mg)	Carb. (g)	Fiber (g)	Prot. (g)	Servings/Exchanges
Sausage Lover's	1 slice	300	17	51	6	0	30	590	27	2	12	1 1/2 starch, 1 high-fat meat, 1 1/2 fat
Super Supreme	1 slice	320	17	47	6	0.5	30	700	28	2	13	2 starch, 1 high-fat meat, 2 fat
Supreme	1 slice	300	16	48	6	0.5	25	600	27	2	12	1 1/2 starch, 2 high-fat meat
Veggie Lover's	1 slice	250	11	39	4	0	15	440	28	2	9	2 starch, 1 high-fat meat

14" LARGE THIN 'N CRISPY PIZZA

	Serving Size	Cal.	Fat (g)	% Cal. Fat	Sat. Fat (g)	Trans Fat (g)	Chol. (mg)	Sod. (mg)	Carb. (g)	Fiber (g)	Prot. (g)	Servings/Exchanges
✔Cheese Only	1 slice	190	8	37	4.5	0.5	25	460	20	1	9	1 starch, 1 high-fat meat
✔Chicken Supreme	1 slice	180	6	30	3	0	20	480	21	1	11	1 1/2 starch, 1 medium-fat meat
Meat Lover's	1 slice	250	13	46	6	0.5	35	700	20	2	12	1 starch, 1 high-fat meat, 1 1/2 fat

(*Continued*)

✔ = Healthiest Bets

14" LARGE THIN 'N CRISPY PIZZA *(Continued)*	Amount	Cal.	Fat (g)	% Cal. Fat	Sat. Fat (g)	Trans Fat (g)	Chol. (mg)	Sod. (mg)	Carb. (g)	Fiber (g)	Pro. (g)	Servings/Exchanges
Pepperoni	1 slice	200	9	40	4.5	0	25	520	19	1	9	1 starch, 1 high-fat meat
Pepperoni Lover's	1 slice	250	14	50	6	0.5	35	660	20	1	12	1 starch, 1 high-fat meat, 1 1/2 fat
✓Quartered Ham	1 slice	170	6	31	3	0	20	500	19	1	9	1 starch, 1 medium-fat meat
Super Supreme	1 slice	240	12	45	5	0.5	30	710	21	2	12	1 1/2 starch, 1 high-fat meat, 1 fat
Supreme	1 slice	220	11	45	5	0.5	25	600	21	2	11	1 1/2 starch, 1 high-fat meat, 1/2 fat
✓Veggie Lover's	1 slice	170	7	37	3	0	15	450	21	2	8	1 1/2 starch, 1 medium-fat meat

14" STUFFED CRUST PIZZA

	Amount											Exchanges
Cheese Only	1 slice	360	13	32	8	0.5	40	920	43	2	18	3 starch, 1 medium-fat meat, 1 fat
Chicken Supreme	1 slice	380	13	30	7	0.5	40	1020	44	3	20	3 starch, 2 medium-fat meat
Meat Lover's	1 slice	450	21	42	10	1	55	1250	43	3	21	3 starch, 2 high-fat meat, 1/2 fat
Pepperoni	1 slice	370	15	36	8	0.5	45	970	42	3	18	3 starch, 1 high-fat meat, 1 1/2 fat
Pepperoni Lover's	1 slice	420	19	40	40	1	55	1120	43	3	21	3 starch, 2 high-fat meat
Quartered Ham	1 slice	340	11	29	6	0.5	40	960	42	2	18	3 starch, 1 medium-fat meat, 1 fat
Super Supreme	1 slice	440	20	40	9	0.5	50	1270	45	3	21	3 starch, 2 high-fat meat, 1/2 fat

✔ = Healthiest Bets

(Continued)

14" STUFFED CRUST PIZZA *(Continued)*	Amount	Cal.	Fat (g)	% Cal. Fat	Sat. Fat (g)	Trans Fat (g)	Chol. (mg)	Sod. (mg)	Carb. (g)	Fiber (g)	Pro. (g)	Servings/Exchanges
Supreme	1 slice	400	16	36	8	0.5	45	1070	44	3	20	3 starch, 2 high-fat meat
Veggie Lover's	1 slice	360	14	35	7	0.5	35	980	45	3	16	3 starch, 1 high-fat meat, 1 fat
16" FULL HOUSE XL PIZZA												
Cheese Only	1 slice	280	12	38	6	0.5	25	760	30	3	12	2 starch, 1 high-fat meat, 1/2 fat
Chicken Supreme	1 slice	270	10	33	4	0	25	770	31	3	13	2 starch, 1 high-fat meat, 1/2 fat
Meat Lover's	1 slice	380	21	49	8	0.5	45	1120	30	3	17	2 starch, 2 high-fat meat, 1 fat
Pepperoni	1 slice	290	13	40	5	0	25	810	30	3	12	2 starch, 1 high-fat meat, 1 fat

	Serving										Exchanges
Pepperoni Lover's	1 slice	310	15	43	6	0.5	30	880	30	3	13	2 starch, 1 high-fat meat, 1 1/2 fat
Quartered Ham	1 slice	260	10	34	4	0	25	790	30	3	12	2 starch, 1 medium-fat meat, 1 fat
Super Supreme	1 slice	330	16	43	6	0.5	35	1000	32	3	15	2 starch, 1 high-fat meat, 1 1/2 fat
Supreme	1 slice	310	15	43	6	0.5	30	890	31	3	13	2 starch, 1 high-fat meat, 1 1/2 fat
Veggie Lover's	1 slice	260	11	38	4	0	20	740	32	3	10	2 starch, 1 medium-fat meat, 1 fat

6" PERSONAL PAN PIZZAS

	Serving										Exchanges
✔Cheese Only	4 slices	630	27	38	12	1	60	1240	71	4	27	4 1/2 starch, 2 high-fat meat, 2 fat
✔Chicken Supreme	4 slices	620	23	33	9	0.5	55	1310	73	4	31	5 starch, 2 medium-fat meat, 2 fat

(Continued)

✔ = Healthiest Bets

6" PERSONAL PAN PIZZA *(Continued)*	Amount	Cal.	Fat (g)	% Cal. Fat	Sat. Fat (g)	Trans Fat (g)	Chol. (mg)	Sod. (mg)	Carb. (g)	Fiber (g)	Pro. (g)	Servings/Exchanges
Meat Lover's	4 slices	800	41	46	16	1	90	1910	71	5	36	4 1/2 starch, 3 high-fat meat, 3 fat
✔Pepperoni	4 slices	660	30	40	12	1	60	1370	70	4	27	4 1/2 starch, 2 high-fat meat, 2 1/2 fat
Pepperoni Lover's	4 slices	800	42	47	17	1	95	1760	71	4	35	4 1/2 starch, 3 high-fat meat, 3 fat
✔Quartered Ham	4 slices	580	22	34	9	0.5	55	1330	70	4	26	4 1/2 starch, 2 lean meat, 3 fat
Super Supreme	4 slices	790	40	45	15	1	85	1940	74	6	35	5 starch, 3 high-fat meat, 2 1/2 fat
Supreme	4 slices	750	36	43	15	1	70	1680	73	6	32	5 starch, 3 high-fat meat, 1 1/2 fat
✔Veggie Lover's	4 slices	580	23	35	9	0.5	40	1150	73	5	22	5 starch, 1 high-fat meat, 2 1/2 fat

APPETIZERS

	Amount	Cal.	Fat (g)	% Fat Cal.	Sat. Fat (g)	Trans Fat (g)	Chol. (mg)	Sod. (mg)	Carb. (g)	Fiber (g)	Prot. (g)	Servings/Exchanges
✔ Breadsticks	1	150	6	36	1	0	0	220	20	0	4	1 1/2 starch, 1 fat
✔ Breadsticks Dipping Sauce	6 T	50	0	0	0	0	0	370	11	2	1	1/2 starch
Cheese Breadsticks	1	200	10	45	3.5	0	15	340	21	0	7	1 1/2 starch, 2 fat
Hot Wings	2 pieces	110	6	49	2	0	70	450	1	0	11	2 lean meat
Mild Wings	2 pieces	110	7	57	2	0	70	320	0	0	11	2 lean meat
Wing Blue Cheese Dipping Sauce	3 T	230	24	93	5	1	25	550	2	0	2	5 fat
Wing Ranch Dipping Sauce	3 T	210	22	94	3.5	0.5	10	340	4	0	2	4 1/2 fat

DESSERTS

	Amount	Cal.	Fat (g)	% Fat Cal.	Sat. Fat (g)	Trans Fat (g)	Chol. (mg)	Sod. (mg)	Carb. (g)	Fiber (g)	Prot. (g)	Servings/Exchanges
Apple Dessert Pizza	1 slice	260	4	13	0.5	0.5	0	250	53	1	4	3 1/2 carb, 1 fat
Cherry Dessert Pizza	1 slice	240	4	15	0.5	0.5	0	250	47	1	4	3 carb, 1 fat
✔ Cinnamon Sticks	2 pieces	170	5	26	1	0	0	170	27	0	4	1 1/2 carb, 1 fat
White Icing Dipping Cup	4 T	190	0	0	0	0	0	0	46	0	0	3 carb

✔ = Healthiest Bets

(*Continued*)

	Amount	Cal.	Fat (g)	% Cal. Fat	Sat. Fat (g)	Trans Fat (g)	Chol. (mg)	Sod. (mg)	Carb. (g)	Fiber (g)	Pro. (g)	Servings/Exchanges
DRESSINGS												
Caesar Dressing	2 T	150	16	96	3	1	5	380	1	0	0	3 fat
French Dressing	2 T	140	11	70	2	0.5	0	220	11	0	0	1/2 carb, 2 fat
Italian Dressing	2 T	140	15	96	2.5	1	0	360	2	0	0	3 fat
✔Lite Italian Dressing	2 T	60	5	75	1	0	0	410	5	0	0	1 fat
✔Lite Ranch Dressing	2 T	70	7	90	1.5	0	10	200	0	0	0	1 1/2 fat
Ranch Dressing	2 T	100	10	90	2	0.5	5	240	2	0	0	2 fat
Thousand Island Dressing	2 T	110	9	73	1.5	1.5	10	300	6	0	0	1/2 carb, 2 fat
FIT 'N DELICIOUS 12" PIZZA												
Diced Chicken, Mushroom, Jalapeño	1 slice	170	5	26	2	0	15	690	22	2	10	1 1/2 starch, 1 lean meat

Item	Serving											Exchanges
✔ Diced Chicken, Red Onion & Green Pepper	1 slice	170	5	26	2	0	15	460	23	2	10	1 1/2 starch, 1 lean meat
✔ Green Pepper, Red Onion, & Diced Red Tomato	1 slice	150	4	24	1.5	0	10	330	22	2	6	1 1/2 starch, 1 lean meat
✔ Ham, Pineapple, & Diced Red Tomato	1 slice	160	4	22	2	0	15	470	24	2	8	1 1/2 starch, 1 fat
✔ Ham, Red Onion, & Mushroom	1 slice	160	5	28	2	0	15	470	22	2	8	1 1/2 starch, 1 fat
Tomato, Mushroom, & Jalapeño	1 slice	150	4	24	2	0	10	590	22	2	6	1 1/2 starch, 1 lean meat
FIT 'N DELICIOUS 14" PIZZA												
Diced Chicken, Mushroom, Jalapeño	1 slice	160	5	28	2	0	15	630	20	2	9	1 1/2 starch, 1 lean meat
✔ Diced Chicken, Red Onion & Green Pepper	1 slice	160	4	22	2	0	15	420	22	2	9	1 1/2 starch, 1 lean meat

✔ = Healthiest Bets

(Continued)

FIT 'N DELICIOUS 14" PIZZA *(Continued)*	Amount	Cal.	Fat (g)	% Cal. Fat	Sat. Fat (g)	Trans Fat (g)	Chol. (mg)	Sod. (mg)	Carb. (g)	Fiber (g)	Pro. (g)	Servings/Exchanges
✔Green Pepper, Red Onion, & Diced Tomato	1 slice	140	3.5	22	1.5	0	10	330	22	2	6	1 1/2 starch, 1/2 fat
✔Ham, Pineapple, & Diced Red Tomato	1 slice	150	4	24	2	0	15	440	22	1	7	1 1/2 starch, 1 lean meat
✔Ham, Red Onion, & Mushroom	1 slice	150	4	24	2	0	15	440	21	2	8	1 1/2 starch, 1 lean meat
Tomato, Mushroom, & Jalapeño	1 slice	140	4	25	1.5	0	10	540	21	2	6	1 1/2 starch, 1 lean meat

✔ = Healthiest Bets

Starbucks

www.starbucks.com

Note: The nutrition information for Starbucks' beverages is based on the information provided on the Starbucks Web site and the standard beverage recipes used across the country. Starbucks notes, however, that the nutrition information for its foods differs from one area of the country to another. For this reason, the nutrition information for foods on the Web site is based on the zip code of individual Starbucks stores. To give you a sense of the nutrition content of Starbucks' foods, this book provides the information from foods served in the Washington, DC, area. The meals below are also based on this information. To get the most precise nutrition information for the items served in the Starbucks you frequent, go to the Web site. You may also be able to get the nutrition information for the foods in the store you visit by asking at the counter.

(*Continued*)

Light & Lean Choice

1 Low-Fat Blueberry Muffin
1 Caffe Latte (12 oz)

Calories	400	Cholesterol (mg)	5
Fat (g)	5	Sodium (mg)	660
% calories from fat	11	Carbohydrate (g)	74
Saturated fat (g)	2	Fiber (g)	1
Trans fat (g)	0	Protein (g)	19

Exchanges: 3 1/2 starch, 1 1/2 fat-free milk

Healthy & Hearty Choice

1 Blueberry Scone
1 Coffee Frappuccino (no whipped cream) (12 oz)

Calories	550	Cholesterol (mg)	50
Fat (g)	18	Sodium (mg)	410
% calories from fat	35	Carbohydrate (g)	88
Saturated fat (g)	8	Fiber (g)	5
Trans fat (g)	0.5	Protein (g)	11

Exchanges: 6 carb, 3 1/2 fat

Starbucks

	Amount	Cal.	Fat (g)	% Cal. Fat	Sat. Fat (g)	Trans Fat (g)	Chol. (mg)	Sod. (mg)	Carb. (g)	Fiber (g)	Pro. (g)	Servings/Exchanges
BAGELS												
✔ Cinnamon Raisin	1	320	1	2	0	0	0	460	70	4	10	4 1/2 starch
✔ Multigrain	1	360	4	10	0	0	0	480	72	6	12	5 starch
✔ Plain	1	320	1	2	0	0	0	480	68	2	10	4 1/2 starch
BROWNIES, BARS, TARTS												
Banana Cha Cha	1	510	31	54	13	2.5	55	200	54	2	5	3 1/2 carb, 6 fat
Banana Crème Bar	1	630	42	60	25	2	70	230	58	3	7	4 carb, 8 fat
Crispy Marshmallow Square	1	360	11	27	4.5	1.5	15	510	67	0	3	4 carb, 2 fat
Mint Brownie	1	480	28	52	13	1	50	140	52	2	4	3 1/2 carb, 5 1/2 fat
Raspberry Bar	1	270	13	43	8	0	35	130	36	1	3	2 1/2 carb, 2 1/2 fat

✔ = Healthiest Bets

(Continued)

BROWNIES, BARS, TARTS *(Continued)*	Amount	Cal.	Fat (g)	% Cal. Fat	Sat. Fat (g)	Trans Fat (g)	Chol. (mg)	Sod. (mg)	Carb. (g)	Fiber (g)	Pro. (g)	Servings/Exchanges
Starbucks Espresso Brownie	1	370	21	51	13	n/a	85	115	43	2	4	3 carb, 4 fat
Toffee Almond Bar	1	430	21	43	7	3.5	50	440	56	1	4	4 carb, 4 fat
CAKES												
Banana Loaf	1	360	18	45	11	0	100	380	47	1	4	3 carb, 3 fat
Chocolate Marble Pound	1	400	21	47	11	0	130	370	49	1	6	3 carb, 4 fat
Crumble Berry Coffee	1	520	26	45	9	4	75	350	69	2	6	4 1/2 carb, 5 fat
Iced Lemon Pound	1	500	23	41	12	0	145	380	69	1	6	4 1/2 carb, 4 1/2 fat
Old Fashioned Crumb	1	670	32	42	15	1	115	360	89	1	8	6 carb, 6 fat
Reduced-Fat Banana Coffee	1 piece	470	15	28	11	1	0	470	77	1	5	5 carb, 3 fat
Reduced-Fat Blueberry Coffee	1 piece	350	11	28	6	1	10	430	61	1	4	4 carb, 2 fat
✓ Reduced-Fat Cinnamon Swirl Coffee	1 piece	330	8	21	4.5	1	5	400	62	1	4	4 carb, 1 1/2 fat

	Amount											
Vanilla Pound	1 piece	430	22	46	11	1	135	380	53	1		3 1/2 carb, 4 fat

COOKIES

Black and White	1	430	17	35	3	0	50	210	68	2	4	4 1/2 carb, 3 1/2 fat
Chocolate Chunk	1	470	23	44	7	5	25	330	62	2	6	4 carb, 4 1/2 fat
Molasses Chew	1	410	12	26	2	4	25	410	67	1	6	4 1/2 carb, 2 fat
Oatmeal Raisin	1	420	15	32	2.5	4.5	30	310	64	3	7	4 carb, 3 fat
Rainbow	1	480	19	35	12	0	55	340	72	1	4	5 carb, 4 fat
Spring Flower	1	400	20	45	11	2	15	190	51	1	4	3 1/2 carb, 4 fat

CROISSANTS, BREADS

Butter Croissant	1	310	16	46	10	0	40	300	35	1	5	2 carb, 3 fat
Cinnamon Nut Crescent	1	320	24	67	12	0	50	230	22	1	5	1 1/2 carb, 5 fat

CUPCAKES

Black Bottom	1	580	29	45	8	1	80	640	72	2	6	5 carb, 6 fat

(Continued)

✔ = Healthiest Bets n/a = not available

CUPCAKES (Continued)	Amount	Cal.	Fat (g)	% Cal. Fat	Sat. Fat (g)	Trans Fat (g)	Chol. (mg)	Sod. (mg)	Carb. (g)	Fiber (g)	Pro. (g)	Servings/Exchanges
Chocolate	1	400	22	49	7	2	10	260	50	2	3	3 carb, 4 fat
Orange	1	310	15	43	5	1.5	5	230	42	1	2	4 carb, 3 fat
Vanilla	1	340	15	39	5	1.5	10	330	48	1	3	3 carb, 3 fat
DOUGHNUTS, SWEET ROLLS, DANISH												
Apple Fritter	1	790	37	42	8	11	55	830	109	11	11	7 carb, 7 fat
Chocolate Glazed Doughnut	1	330	19	51	5	5	0	320	36	2	4	2 1/2 carb, 4 fat
Cinnamon Twist	1	320	17	47	1.5	5	25	280	37	1	4	2 1/2 carb, 3 fat
Cream Cheese Danish	1	590	34	51	10	7	35	750	60	1	11	4 carb, 7 fat
Glazed Doughnut	1	350	19	48	5	5	0	330	41	1	5	3 carb, 4 fat
FRAPPUCCINO BLENDED COFFEES												
Caffe Vanilla w/ whipped cream	12 oz	250	10	36	6	0	40	230	36	3	5	2 carb, 2 fat

Item												
Caffe Vanilla w/out whipped cream	12 oz	160	1	5	0	0	0	220	34	3	5	2 carb
Caramel Frappuccino w/ whipped cream	12 oz	240	10	37	6	0	40	230	31	2	5	1 carb, 1 milk, 2 fat
✔Caramel Frappuccino w/out whipped cream	12 oz	140	1.5	9	0	0	5	220	28	2	5	1 carb, 1/2 milk
Coffee Frappuccino w/ whipped cream	12 oz	200	10	45	6	0	40	230	23	2	5	1 1/2 carb, 2 fat
✔Coffee Frappuccino w/out whipped cream	12 oz	110	1	8	0	0	0	220	22	2	5	1 1/2 carb
Mocha Frappuccino w/ whipped cream	12 oz	230	10	39	6	0	40	230	29	3	5	2 carb, 2 fat
✔Mocha Frappuccino w/out whipped cream	12 oz	140	2	12	0	0	0	220	28	3	5	2 carb

✔ = Healthiest Bets

(Continued)

	Amount	Cal.	Fat (g)	% Cal. Fat	Sat. Fat (g)	Trans Fat (g)	Chol. (mg)	Sod. (mg)	Carb. (g)	Fiber (g)	Pro. (g)	Servings/Exchanges
FRAPPUCCINO BLENDED CREMES												
Double Chocolate Chip w/ whipped cream	12 oz	430	17	35	10	0	40	300	60	2	12	3 carb, 1 milk, 3 fat
Double Chocolate Chip w/out whipped cream	12 oz	330	8	21	4	0	4	300	57	2	12	3 carb, 1 milk, 1 fat
Tazo Chai w/ whipped cream	12 oz	370	12	29	7	0	40	280	54	0	10	3 carb, 1 milk, 2 fat
✔Tazo Chai w/out whipped cream	12 oz	280	3.5	11	1	0	4	270	52	0	10	3 carb, 1 milk, 1/2 fat
Vanilla Bean w/ whipped cream	12 oz	370	12	29	7	0.5	40	270	52	0	10	3 carb, 1 milk, 2 fat
✔Vanilla Bean w/out whipped cream	12 oz	270	3.5	11	1	0	4	270	51	0	10	3 carb, 1 milk, 1 fat

FRAPPUCCINO JUICE BLEND

	Serving	Calories	Fat (g)	% Fat Cal	Sat Fat (g)	Chol (mg)	Sodium (mg)	Carb (g)	Fiber (g)	Protein (g)	Exchanges
Pomegranate	12 oz	210	0	0	0	0	10	51	1	2	3 1/2 fruit
Tangerine	12 oz	140	0	0	0	0	20	34	1	1	2 fruit

ICED COFFEES

	Serving	Calories	Fat (g)	% Fat Cal	Sat Fat (g)	Chol (mg)	Sodium (mg)	Carb (g)	Fiber (g)	Protein (g)	Exchanges
✔ Iced Caffe Americano	12 oz	10	0	0	0	0	10	2	0	1	free
✔ Iced Caffe Latte	12 oz	70	0	0	0	4	105	11	0	7	1 milk
Iced Caffe Mocha w/ whipped cream	12 oz	230	10	39	6	40	85	28	1	7	2 carb, 2 fat
✔ Iced Caffe Mocha w/out whipped cream	12 oz	130	2	13	0	4	80	27	1	7	1 1/2 carb
✔ Iced Syrup Flavored Latte	12 oz	120	0	0	0	0	90	24	0	6	1 1/2 carb
✔ Iced Vanilla Latte	12 oz	120	0	0	0	0	90	24	0	6	1/2 carb, 1 milk
Iced White Chocolate Mocha w/ whipped cream	12 oz	330	13	35	9	40	170	44	0	9	3 carb, 2 1/2 fat

✔ = Healthiest Bets

(Continued)

ICED COFFEES *(Continued)*	Amount	Cal.	Fat (g)	% Cal. Fat	Sat. Fat (g)	Trans Fat (g)	Chol. (mg)	Sod. (mg)	Carb. (g)	Fiber (g)	Pro. (g)	Servings/Exchanges
Iced White Chocolate Mocha 12 oz w/out whipped cream	12 oz	240	4	15	3.5	0	4	170	42	0	9	3 carb, 1 fat
MUFFINS												
Blueberry	1	420	20	42	4	1	65	380	55	1	5	4 carb, 4 fat
Carrot Walnut	1	510	29	51	6	0	70	400	55	3	6	4 carb, 6 fat
Chocolate Cream Cheese	1	430	26	54	6	0	75	380	48	1	5	3 carb, 5 fat
Lemon Poppyseed	1	440	23	47	5	0	85	400	52	1	6	3 1/2 carb, 4 1/2 fat
✓Lowfat Blueberry	1	280	5	16	2	0	5	490	56	1	7	4 carb, 1 fat
PIES, TARTS												
White Chocolate Strawberry Torte	1	620	34	49	16	n/a	65	200	76	1	5	5 carb, 7 fat

SCONES

Blueberry	1	410	16	35	8	0.5	45	190	60	3	6	4 carb, 3 fat
Cinnamon	1	460	19	37	9	3	50	190	66	1	5	4 1/2 carb, 4 fat
Maple Oat Nut	1	430	16	33	7	0	40	370	67	2	6	4 1/2 carb, 3 fat
Reduced-Fat Lemon	1	410	13	28	7	0	45	290	65	3	6	4 carb, 3 fat
SPECIALTY BEVERAGES												
Caramel Apple Cider w/ whipped cream	12 oz	320	8	22	5	n/a	35	25	59	0	0	4 carb, 1 1/2 fat
Caramel Apple Cider w/out whipped cream	12 oz	230	0	0	0	n/a	0	15	55	0	0	3 1/2 carb
Chantico Drinking Chocolate	6 oz	390	21	48	10	n/a	25	105	51	6	11	3 carb, 1 milk, 3 fat
Chocolate Milk	12 oz	190	1.5	7	0	n/a	5	170	35	1	13	1 1/2 carb, 1 milk
Cinnamon Dolce Crème w/ whipped cream	12 oz	270	8	26	5	0.5	40	180	37	0	12	1 1/2 carb, 1 milk, 1 1/2 fat

✔ = Healthiest Bets   n/a = not available

(Continued)

SPECIALTY BEVERAGES *(Continued)*	Amount	Cal.	Fat (g)	% Cal. Fat	Sat. Fat (g)	Trans Fat (g)	Chol. (mg)	Sod. (mg)	Carb. (g)	Fiber (g)	Pro. (g)	Servings/Exchanges
Hot Chocolate w/ whipped cream	12 oz	290	9	27	5	0.5	35	160	41	1	12	1 1/2 carb, 1 milk ,2 fat
Hot Chocolate w/out whipped cream	12 oz	210	2	8	0	0.5	5	150	40	1	12	1 1/2 carb, 1 milk, 1/2 fat
Steamed Apple Cider	12 oz	180	0	0	0	n/a	0	15	45	0	0	3 carb
Vanilla Crème w/ whipped cream	12 oz	260	8	27	5	0.5	35	170	33	0	11	1 carb, 1 milk ,1 1/2 fat
✓Vanilla Crème w/out whipped cream	12 oz	180	0	0	0	0.5	4	170	32	0	11	1 carb, 1 milk
White Hot Chocolate w/ whipped cream	12 oz	380	12	28	8	0.5	40	260	52	0	15	2 1/2 carb, 1 milk, 2 1/2 fat
White Hot Chocolate w/out whipped cream	12 oz	300	5	15	3.5	0.5	10	250	51	0	15	2 1/2 carb, 1 milk, 1/2 fat

SPECIALTY COFFEES

✔ Café Mistro/Café Au Lait	12 oz	60	0	0	0	0	4	90	9	0	6
✔ Caffe Americano	12 oz	10	0	0	0	n/a	0	0	0	2	0
✔ Caffe Latte	12 oz	120	0	0	0	0	5	170	18	0	12
Caffe Mocha w/ whipped cream	12 oz	260	9	31	5	35	140	34	1	11	
Caffe Mocha w/out whipped cream	12 oz	170	2	10	0	5	135	33	1	11	
✔ Cappuccino	12 oz	80	0	0	0	4	100	11	0	7	
✔ Caramel Mocchiato w/out whipped cream	12 oz	170	2	10	0	5	160	30	0	11	
Syrup Flavored Latte	12 oz	170	0	0	0	4	280	33	0	11	
Toffee Nut Latte w/ whipped cream	12 oz	260	8	27	5	n/a	270	32	0	11	

Exchanges:
- Café Mistro/Café Au Lait: 1 milk
- Caffe Americano: 1 free
- Caffe Latte: 1 1/2 milk
- Caffe Mocha w/ whipped cream: 1 1/2 carb, 1 milk, 2 fat
- Caffe Mocha w/out whipped cream: 1 1/2 carb, 1 milk
- Cappuccino: 1 milk
- Caramel Mocchiato w/out whipped cream: 1 carb, 1 milk, 1/2 fat
- Syrup Flavored Latte: 1 carb, 1 milk
- Toffee Nut Latte w/ whipped cream: 1 carb, 1 milk, 2 fat

✔ = Healthiest Bets   n/a = not available

(Continued)

SPECIALTY COFFEES (Continued)	Amount	Cal.	Fat (g)	% Cal. Fat	Sat. Fat (g)	Trans Fat (g)	Chol. (mg)	Sod. (mg)	Carb. (g)	Fiber (g)	Pro. (g)	Servings/Exchanges
Toffee Nut Latte w/out whipped cream	12 oz	180	0	0	0	n/a	5	270	32	0	11	1 carb, 1 milk
✔Vanilla Latte	12 oz	170	0	0	0	0	4	150	31	0	11	1 carb, 1 milk
White Chocolate Mocha w/ whipped cream	12 oz	340	11	29	8	0	40	220	46	0	12	2 carb, 1 milk, 2 fat
White Chocolate Mocha w/out whipped cream	12 oz	260	4	13	3	0	5	210	45	0	12	2 carb, 1 milk, 1 fat
TAZO TEA												
✔Tazo Black Iced Tea	12 oz	60	0	0	0	0	0	5	16	0	0	1 carb
✔Tazo Black Tea Lemonade	12 oz	90	0	0	0	0	0	15	23	0	0	1 1/2 carb
Tazo Chai Iced Tea Latte	12 oz	170	0	0	0	0	5	90	36	0	6	2 carb
Tazo Chai Tea Latte	12 oz	170	0	0	0	0	5	95	37	0	6	2 carb

✓Tazo Green Iced Tea	12 oz	60	0	0	0	0	0	5	16	0	0	1 carb
✓Tazo Green Tea Lemonade	12 oz	90	0	0	0	0	0	15	23	0	0	1 1/2 carb
✓Tazo Passion Iced Tea	12 oz	60	0	0	0	0	0	5	16	0	0	1 carb
✓Tazo Passion Tea Lemonade	12 oz	90	0	0	0	0	0	15	23	0	0	1 1/2 carb

✔ = Healthiest Bets

Subway

www.subway.com

Light & Lean Choice

1 Minestrone Soup (10 oz)
1 Grilled Chicken and Baby Spinach Salad
Fat-free Vinaigrette (2 T or 1/2 serving)
1 Oatmeal Raisin Cookie

Calories......................448	Cholesterol (mg).........69
Fat (g) 12	Sodium (mg)..........1,890
% calories from fat ...24	Carbohydrate (g).........62
Saturated fat (g) 3.5	Fiber (g).....................9
Trans fat (g)............2.5	Protein (g) 27

Exchanges: 2 starch, 2 carb, 2 vegetable, 3 lean meat, 1 fat

Healthy & Hearty Choice

1 Minestrone Soup (10 oz)
1 Turkey Breast and Ham Sandwich (6")
1 Oatmeal Raisin Cookie

Calories......................580	Cholesterol (mg).........44
Fat (g) 14	Sodium (mg)..........2,310
Saturated fat (g) 22	Carbohydrate (g).........94
Saturated fat (g) 4	Fiber (g).....................9
Trans fat (g)............2.5	Protein (g) 37

Exchanges: 5 starch, 2 carb, 1 vegetable, 3 lean meat, 2 fat

(Continued)

Subway

6" DOUBLE MEAT SUBS

	Amount	Cal.	Fat (g)	% Cal. Fat	Sat. Fat (g)	Trans Fat (g)	Chol. (mg)	Sod. (mg)	Carb. (g)	Fiber (g)	Pro. (g)	Servings/Exchanges
DM Cheese Steak	1	450	14	28	6	0	60	1470	50	6	37	3 starch, 4 lean meat
DM Chipotle Southwest Cheese Steak	1	540	24	40	7	0	70	1680	51	7	37	3 1/2 starch, 4 medium-fat meat
DM Classic Tuna	1	790	55	62	11	1	80	1340	45	4	32	3 starch, 3 lean meat, 8 1/2 fat
DM Cold Cut Combo	1	550	28	45	10	1	110	2380	49	4	31	3 starch, 3 high-fat meat, 1/2 fat
DM Ham	1	380	7	16	2.5	0	50	2180	57	4	28	3 1/2 starch, 2 lean meat
DM Italian BMT	1	630	35	50	14	0	100	2890	49	4	34	3 starch, 3 high-fat meat, 2 fat

DM Meatball Marinara	1	960	42	39	18	2	85	2490	82	10	37	5 1/2 starch, 3 high-fat meat, 4 fat
DM Oven Roasted Chicken	1	430	8	16	2	0	90	1520	50	4	39	3 1/2 starch, 3 lean meat
DM Roast Beef	1	360	7	17	3.5	0	40	1320	46	4	29	3 starch, 3 lean meat
DM Seafood Sensation	1	640	38	53	8	1	40	1580	58	5	20	3 1/2 starch, 1 medium-fat meat, 6 1/2 fat
DM Subway Club	1	420	8	17	3.5	0	65	2100	50	4	39	3 starch, 4 lean meat
DM Sweet Onion Chicken Teriyaki	1	490	7	12	2	0	100	1630	68	4	43	4 1/2 starch, 4 lean meat
DM Turkey Breast	1	340	6	15	1.5	0	40	1520	48	4	28	3 starch, 3 very-lean meat
DM Turkey Breast & Ham	1	360	7	17	2	0	50	1950	50	4	31	3 1/2 starch, 3 lean meat
DM Turkey Breast, Ham & Bacon Melt	1	500	17	30	8	0	82	2520	51	4	40	3 1/2 starch, 4 lean meat, 1/2 fat

✔ = Healthiest Bets

(Continued)

6" SANDWICHES

	Amount	Cal.	Fat (g)	% Cal. Fat	Sat. Fat (g)	Trans Fat (g)	Chol. (mg)	Sod. (mg)	Carb. (g)	Fiber (g)	Pro. (g)	Servings/Exchanges
Absolute Angus Steak	1	420	20	42	8	n/a	70	730	44	4	20	3 starch, 2 medium-fat meat, 1 1/2 fat
Barbecue Chicken	1	310	6	17	2	0	35	1110	52	5	16	3 1/2 starch, 2 lean meat
Barbecue Rib Patty	1	420	19	40	6	0	50	830	47	4	20	3 starch, 1 high-fat meat, 2 fat
BBQ Steak & Monterey Cheddar Cheese	1	390	11	25	5	0	40	1290	53	6	26	3 1/2 starch, 2 lean meat, 1/2 fat
Big Hot Pastrami	1	580	30	46	10	0	15	1880	48	4	33	3 starch, 3 high-fat meat, 1 fat
Buffalo Chicken	1	390	13	30	3	0	55	1510	46	5	26	3 starch, 2 lean meat, 1 1/2 fat

Item	Serving											Exchanges
Cheese Steak	1	360	10	25	4.5	0	35	1090	47	5	24	3 starch, 2 medium-fat meat
Chicken & Bacon Ranch	1	530	25	42	10	0.5	90	1440	47	5	36	3 starch, 4 medium-fat meat
Chicken Parmesan	1	510	18	31	6	0	38	1410	64	5	26	4 starch, 2 medium-fat meat, 1 fat
Chipotle Chicken & Bacon Cheese Melt	1	560	27	43	10	0	95	1410	47	5	36	3 starch, 4 medium-fat meat
Chipotle Southwest Cheese Steak	1	450	20	40	6	0	45	1310	48	6	24	3 starch, 2 medium-fat meat, 2 fat
Classic Tuna	1	530	31	52	7	0.5	45	1030	45	4	22	3 starch, 2 lean meat, 4 fat
Cold Cut Combo	1	410	17	37	7	0.5	60	1550	47	4	21	3 starch, 2 high-fat meat

(Continued)

✔ = Healthiest Bets   n/a = not available

6" SANDWICHES *(Continued)*	Amount	Cal.	Fat (g)	% Cal. Fat	Sat. Fat (g)	Trans Fat (g)	Chol. (mg)	Sod. (mg)	Carb. (g)	Fiber (g)	Pro. (g)	Servings/Exchanges
✔Gardenburger	1	390	7	16	2.5	0	5	970	66	9	19	4 starch, 1 lean meat, 1/2 fat
Garlic Lover's Roast Beef Cheese Melt	1	510	25	44	10	0	60	1280	48	5	26	3 starch, 2 medium-fat meat, 3 fat
Ham	1	290	5	15	1.5	0	25	1280	47	4	18	3 starch, 1 lean meat
Italian BMT	1	450	21	42	8	0	55	1790	47	4	23	3 starch, 2 high-fat meat
Meatball Marinara	1	560	24	38	11	1	45	1610	63	7	24	4 starch, 2 medium-fat meat, 2 fat
✔Oven Roasted Chicken Breast	1	330	5	13	1.5	0	45	1020	47	4	24	3 starch, 2 lean meat
Pastrami	1	570	29	45	9	0	10	1890	49	5	32	3 starch, 2 high-fat meat, 2 1/2 fat
✔Roast Beef	1	290	5	15	2	0	20	920	45	4	19	3 starch, 1 lean meat

Spicy Italian	1	480	25	46	9	0	55	1670	46	4	21	3 starch, 2 high-fat meat, 2 fat
Subway Club	1	320	6	16	2	0	35	1310	47	1	24	3 starch, 2 lean meat
Subway Melt	1	382	12	28	5	0	45	1610	48	4	25	3 starch, 2 medium-fat meat
Subway Seafood Sensation	1	450	22	44	6	0.5	25	1150	51	5	16	3 1/2 starch, 1 medium-fat meat, 2 fat
Sweet Onion Chicken Teriyaki	1	370	5	12	1.5	0	50	1220	59	4	26	4 starch, 2 very lean meat
Tuna Double Cheese Melt	1	640	40	56	12	1	75	1210	46	5	28	3 starch, 2 lean meat, 5 1/2 fat
✔Turkey Breast	1	280	5	16	1.5	0	20	1020	46	4	18	3 starch, 1 lean meat
Turkey Breast & Ham	1	290	5	15	1.5	0	25	1230	47	4	20	3 starch, 1 lean meat
Turkey Pastrami	1	330	6	16	1.5	0	10	1500	45	5	26	3 starch, 2 very lean meat

(Continued)

✔ = Healthiest Bets

6" SANDWICHES *(Continued)*	Amount	Cal.	Fat (g)	% Cal. Fat	Sat. Fat (g)	Trans Fat (g)	Chol. (mg)	Sod. (mg)	Carb. (g)	Fiber (g)	Pro. (g)	Servings/Exchanges
Turkey, Bacon & Roasted Garlic Cheese	1	540	28	46	10	0.5	71	1550	49	5	29	3 starch, 3 high-fat meat
✓Veggie Delite	1	230	3	11	1	0	0	520	44	4	9	2 1/2 starch, 1 veg
✓Veggi-Max	1	390	8	18	1.5	0	10	1040	56	7	24	3 1/2 starch, 1 veg, 2 lean meat
BREADS												
✓6" Wheat Bread	1	200	3	13	1	0	0	360	40	3	8	2 1/2 starch
✓6" Hearty Italian Bread	1	210	3	12	1.5	0	0	340	41	3	8	3 starch
✓6" Honey Oat Bread	1	250	4	14	1	0	0	380	48	4	10	3 starch
✓6" Italian White Bread	1	200	3	13	1.5	0	0	340	38	3	7	2 1/2 starch
✓6" Monterey Cheddar Bread	1	240	6	22	3.5	0.5	10	400	39	3	10	2 1/2 starch, 1 fat
✓6" Parmesan Oregano Bread	1	210	4	17	1.5	0.5	0	500	40	3	8	3 starch

	Amount	Cal	Fat (g)	% Cal Fat	Sat Fat (g)	Trans Fat (g)	Chol (mg)	Sod (mg)	Carb (g)	Fiber (g)	Pro (g)	Exchanges/Choices
✔Carb Conscious Wrap	1	120	5	37	0.5	0	0	680	13	8	14	1 starch, 1 lean meat
✔Deli Style Roll	1	170	3	15	1	0	0	280	32	3	6	2 starch
BREAKFAST SANDWICHES ON BREAD												
✔Cheese	1	310	9	26	3.5	0	15	740	43	3	19	3 starch, 1 medium-fat meat
Chipotle Steak & Cheese	1	510	25	44	9	0.5	50	1270	46	4	30	3 starch, 3 medium-fat meat, 1 1/2 fat
Double Bacon & Cheese	1	500	23	41	12	0.5	60	1400	45	4	31	3 starch, 3 high-fat meat, 2 fat
Honey Mustard Ham & Egg	1	310	5	14	1.5	0	15	1150	50	3	20	3 starch, 1 medium-fat meat
Western w/ Cheese	1	400	14	31	7	0	40	1210	46	4	27	3 starch, 2 medium-fat meat, 1/2 fat
BREAKFAST SANDWICHES ON DELI ROUND												
✔Cheese	1	270	9	30	4	0	15	670	35	3	16	2 starch, 1 high-fat meat

(Continued)

✔ = Healthiest Bets

BREAKFAST SANDWICHES ON DELI ROUND *(Continued)*	Amount	Cal.	Fat (g)	% Cal. Fat	Sat. Fat (g)	Trans Fat (g)	Chol. (mg)	Sod. (mg)	Carb. (g)	Fiber (g)	Pro. (g)	Servings/Exchanges
Chipotle Steak & Cheese	1	470	25	47	9	0.5	50	1200	38	4	28	2 1/2 starch, 3 medium-fat meat, 1 1/2 fat
Double Bacon & Cheese	1	460	23	45	12	0.5	60	1320	37	3	29	2 1/2 starch, 3 high-fat meat
✔Honey Mustard Ham & Egg	1	270	5	16	1.5	0	15	1080	42	3	18	3 starch, 1 lean meat
Western w/ Cheese	1	360	14	35	7	0	40	1140	38	3	25	2 1/2 starch, 2 medium-fat meat, 1/2 fat
BREAKFAST WRAPS												
Cheese	1	220	10	40	3.5	0	15	1040	16	8	24	1 starch, 3 lean meat
Chipotle Steak & Cheese	1	430	27	56	8	0	50	1600	19	9	36	1 starch, 5 medium-fat meat
Double Bacon & Cheese	1	420	25	53	11	0.5	60	1720	18	8	37	1 starch, 4 medium-fat meat, 1 fat

Honey Mustard Ham & Egg	1	230	7	27	1	0	15	1480	23	8	26	1 1/2 starch, 3 very lean meat, 1 fat
Western w/ Cheese	1	310	16	46	6	0	40	1540	19	8	32	1 starch, 4 lean meat, 1/2 fat

CHEESE

✓American	for 6" sub	40	4	90	2	0	10	200	1	0	2	1 fat
✓Natural Cheddar	for 6" sub	60	5	75	3	0	15	95	0	0	4	1 medium-fat meat
✓Pepperjack	for 6" sub	50	4	72	2.5	0	15	140	0	0	3	1 fat
✓Provolone	for 6" sub	50	4	72	2	0	10	125	0	0	4	1 fat
✓Shredded Monterey Cheddar	for 6" sub	50	5	90	3	0	15	90	0	0	3	1 fat
✓Swiss	for 6" sub	50	5	90	2.5	0	15	30	0	0	4	1 fat

DELI STYLE SANDWICHES

✓Ham	1	210	4	17	1.5	0	10	770	36	3	11	2 starch, 1 lean meat

(Continued)

✓ = Healthiest Bets

DELI STYLE SANDWICHES *(Continued)*	Amount	Cal.	Fat (g)	% Cal. Fat	Sat. Fat (g)	Trans Fat (g)	Chol. (mg)	Sod. (mg)	Carb. (g)	Fiber (g)	Pro. (g)	Servings/Exchanges
✓Roast Beef	1	220	4.5	18	2	0	15	660	35	3	13	2 starch, 1 medium-fat meat
✓Tuna w/ cheese	1	350	18	46	5	0.5	30	750	35	3	14	2 starch, 2 high-fat meat
✓Turkey Breast	1	210	3.5	15	1.5	0	15	730	36	3	13	2 starch, 1 lean meat
DESSERTS – COOKIES												
✓Chocolate Chip	1	210	10	42	4	1	15	160	30	1	2	2 carb, 1 1/2 fat
✓Chocolate Chunk	1	220	10	40	3.5	2.5	10	105	30	1	2	2 carb, 1 1/2 fat
✓Double Chocolate Chip	1	210	10	42	4	1	15	170	30	1	2	2 carb, 1 1/2 fat
✓M&M Cookie	1	210	10	42	3.5	2.5	15	105	30	1	2	2 carb, 1 1/2 fat
✓Oatmeal Raisin	1	200	8	36	2.5	2.5	15	170	30	2	3	2 carb, 1 1/2 fat
Peanut Butter	1	220	12	49	4	1	10	200	26	1	4	1 1/2 carb, 2 fat

Sugar Cookie	1	230	12	46	3.5	3.5	15	135	28	0	2	2 carb, 2 fat
White Chip Macadamia Nut	1	220	11	45	3.5	1	15	160	28	1	2	2 carb, 2 fat

DESSERTS – PIE

✓ Apple Pie	1 serving	245	10	36	2	n/a	0	290	37	1	0	2 1/2 carb, 1 1/2 fat

FRUIT ROLL UP

Fruit Roll Up	1	50	1	18	0	0	0	55	12	0	0	1 carb

FRUIZIE EXPRESS

✓ Berry Lishus	small	110	0	0	0	0	0	30	28	1	1	2 carb
Berry Lishus w/ banana	small	140	0	0	0	0	0	30	35	2	1	2 carb
✓ Peach Pizzazz	small	100	0	0	0	0	0	25	26	0	0	1 1/2 carb
Pineapple Delight	small	130	0	0	0	0	0	25	33	1	1	2 carb
Pineapple Delight w/ banana	small	160	0	0	0	0	0	25	40	1	1	2 1/2 carb

✓ = Healthiest Bets   n/a = not available

(Continued)

FRUIZIE EXPRESS *(Continued)*	Amount	Cal.	Fat (g)	% Cal. Fat	Sat. Fat (g)	Trans Fat (g)	Chol. (mg)	Sod. (mg)	Carb. (g)	Fiber (g)	Pro. (g)	Servings/Exchanges
✓Sunrise Refresher	small	120	0	0	0	0	0	20	29	1	1	2 carb
SALAD DRESSING												
✓Atkins Honey Mustard	4 T	200	22	99	3	0	0	510	1	0	1	4 1/2 fat
✓Fat Free Italian	4 T	35	0	0	0	0	0	720	7	0	1	1/2 carb
✓Ranch	4 T	200	22	99	3.5	0	10	550	1	0	1	4 1/2 fat
SALADS W/OUT DRESSING & CROUTONS												
✓Grilled Chicken & Baby Spinach	1	140	3	19	1	0	50	450	11	4	20	2 veg, 3 very-lean meat
✓Subway Club	1	160	4	22	1.5	0	35	880	15	4	18	3 veg, 2 very-lean meat
Tuna w/ cheese	1	360	29	72	6	0.5	45	600	12	4	16	2 veg, 2 lean meat, 4 1/2 fat
✓Veggie Delite	1	60	1	15	0	0	0	90	12	4	3	2 veg

SANDWICH CONDIMENTS

	Serving											
Bacon (2 strips)	for 6" sub	45	4	80	1.5	0	10	180	0	0	3	1 fat
Chipotle Southwest Sauce	for 6" sub	100	10	90	1.5	0	10	220	0	0		2 fat
✔Fat Free Honey Mustard	for 6" sub	30	0	0	0	0	0	140	7	0		1/2 carb
✔Fat Free Red Wine Vinaigrette	for 6" sub	30	0	0	0	0	0	340	6	0		1/2 carb
✔Fat Free Sweet Onion Sauce	for 6" sub	40	0	0	0	0	0	100	9	0		1/2 carb
✔Light Mayonnaise	for 6" sub	50	5	90	1	0	10	100	1	0		1 fat
Mayonnaise	for 6" sub	110	12	98	2	0	10	80	0	0		2 1/2 fat
✔Mustard	for 6" sub	5	0	0	0	0	0	115	1	0		free
✔Olive Oil Blend	for 6" sub	45	5	100	0	0	0	0	0	0		1 fat

✔ = Healthiest Bets

(Continued)

SANDWICH CONDIMENTS *(Continued)*	Amount	Cal.	Fat (g)	% Cal. Fat	Sat. Fat (g)	Trans Fat (g)	Chol. (mg)	Sod. (mg)	Carb. (g)	Fiber (g)	Pro. (g)	Servings/Exchanges
Ranch Dressing	for 6" sub	70	8	100	0	0	5	210	0	0	0	1 1/2 fat
✔Vinegar	for 6" sub	0	0	0	0	0	0	0	0	0	0	free
SOUP												
Brown & Wild Rice w/ Chicken	10 oz	230	11	43	3.5	0	50	1170	26	1	6	1 1/2 starch, 2 1/2 fat
Chicken & Dumpling	10 oz	140	3.5	22	1.5	0	5	1230	20	2	7	1 starch, 1 lean meat
Chili Con Carne	10 oz	340	11	29	5	0	60	1100	35	10	20	1 starch, 2 medium-fat meat, 1/2 fat
✔Cream of Broccoli	10 oz	140	5	32	2	0	10	960	18	4	6	1 starch, 1 fat
✔Cream of Potato w/ Bacon	10 oz	220	10	40	4	0	15	980	28	5	5	2 starch, 1 1/2 fat
Golden Broccoli & Cheese	10 oz	180	11	55	4	0	25	990	16	4	5	1 starch, 2 fat
✔Minestrone	10 oz	90	1	10	0	0	4	910	17	3	4	1 starch

	Amount	Calories	Fat (g)	% Cal. Fat	Sat. Fat (g)	Trans Fat (g)	Chol. (mg)	Sodium (mg)	Carb. (g)	Fiber (g)	Protein (g)	Exchanges/Choices
New England Style Clam Chowder	10 oz	150	5	30	1.5	0	10	1400	20	2	5	1/2 starch, 1 milk, 1 fat
Roasted Chicken Noodle	10 oz	90	2	20	0.5	0	20	1130	12	1	6	1 starch
✔ Spanish Style Chicken w/ Rice	10 oz	110	2.5	20	1	0	5	980	16	1	6	1 starch, 1/2 fat
Tomato Garden Vegetable w/ Rotini	10 oz	90	0.5	5	0	0	0	1040	20	3	3	1 starch
Vegetable Beef	10 oz	100	1.5	13	0.5	0	10	1060	17	3	5	1 starch
W R A P S												
Chicken & Bacon Ranch w/ cheese	1	440	27	55	10	0.5	90	1670	18	9	41	1 starch, 5 medium-fat meat
Tuna w/ cheese	1	440	32	65	6	0.5	45	1310	16	9	27	1 starch, 3 lean meat, 4 1/2 fat
Turkey Breast	1	190	6	28	1	0	20	1290	18	9	24	1 starch, 3 very-lean meat
Turkey Breast & Bacon Melt w/ chipotle sauce	1	380	24	56	7	0	50	1780	20	9	31	1 starch, 4 medium-fat meat, 1/2 fat

✔ = Healthiest Bets

Taco Bell

www.tacobell.com

Light & Lean Choice

**1 Soft Beef Taco
1 Tostada
1 Pintos 'n Cheese**

Calories......................590	Cholesterol (mg).........40
Fat (g) 23	Sodium (mg)..........1,990
% calories from fat ...35	Carbohydrate (g).........71
Saturated fat (g) 8.5	Fiber (g)...................14
Trans fat (g)...............3	Protein (g) 28

Exchanges: 4 1/2 starch, 1 vegetable, 2 lean meat, 2 1/2 fat

Healthy & Hearty Choice

**1 Gordita Supreme Chicken
1 Grilled Steak Soft Taco
1 Pintos 'n Cheese**

Calories......................640	Cholesterol (mg).........75
Fat (g) 24	Sodium (mg)..........1,790
% calories from fat ...34	Carbohydrate (g).........69
Saturated fat (g) 10	Fiber (g).....................9
Trans fat (g)............1.5	Protein (g) 38

Exchanges: 4 starch, 1 vegetable, 3 lean meat, 3 fat

(Continued)

Taco Bell

BIG BELL VALUE MENU ITEMS	Amount	Cal.	Fat (g)	% Cal. Fat	Sat. Fat (g)	Trans Fat (g)	Chol. (mg)	Sod. (mg)	Carb. (g)	Fiber (g)	Pro. (g)	Servings/Exchanges
1/2 lb Bean Burrito Especial	1	600	21	31	5	3	15	1760	82	12	21	5 1/2 starch, 1 lean meat, 3 1/2 fat
1/2 lb Beef & Potato Burrito	1	540	25	41	8	3.5	30	1660	66	4	15	4 1/2 starch, 1 medium-fat meat, 2 1/2 fat
1/2 lb Beef Combo Burrito	1	470	19	36	7	2	45	1620	52	5	22	3 1/2 starch, 2 medium-fat meat, 1 fat
Caramel Apple Empanada	1	290	15	46	3.5	3	4	300	37	1	2	2 1/2 starch, 2 1/2 fat
Cheesy Fiesta Potatoes	1	290	18	55	6	3	15	790	28	2	4	2 starch, 3 fat
Double Decker Taco	1	340	14	37	5	1.5	25	810	39	5	14	2 1/2 starch, 1 medium-fat meat, 1 1/2 fat

Grande Soft Taco	1	450	21	42	8	2.5	45	1410	44	2	19	3 starch, 1 medium-fat meat, 3 fat
Spicy Chicken Burrito	1	430	19	39	4.5	2	30	1160	50	4	14	3 1/2 starch, 1 medium-fat meat, 2 fat
✔Spicy Chicken Soft Taco	1	180	7	35	2	0.5	20	580	21	2	10	1 1/2 starch, 1 medium-fat meat

BURRITOS

7-Layer	1	530	21	35	8	2.5	25	1400	66	10	18	4 1/2 starch, 4 fat
Bean	1	370	10	24	3.5	2	10	1200	55	8	14	3 1/2 starch, 2 fat
Chili Cheese	1	390	18	41	9	1.5	40	1080	40	3	16	2 1/2 starch, 1 high-fat meat, 2 fat
Fiesta - Beef	1	390	15	34	5	2	25	1210	50	3	14	3 1/2 starch, 2 1/2 fat
Fiesta - Chicken	1	370	11	26	3.5	1.5	30	1140	49	3	18	3 starch, 1 medium-fat meat, 1 fat

(Continued)

✔ = Healthiest Bets

BURRITOS *(Continued)*	Amount	Cal.	Fat (g)	% Cal. Fat	Sat. Fat (g)	Trans Fat (g)	Chol. (mg)	Sod. (mg)	Carb. (g)	Fiber (g)	Pro. (g)	Servings/Exchanges
Fiesta - Steak	1	370	13	31	4	1.5	25	1140	49	3	16	3 starch, 1 medium-fat meat, 1 1/2 fat
Grilled Stuffed - Beef	1	720	33	41	11	3	55	2140	80	7	27	5 starch, 2 medium-fat meat, 4 fat
Grilled Stuffed - Chicken	1	670	25	33	7	2.5	70	2010	77	7	35	5 starch, 3 medium-fat meat, 1 1/2 fat
Grilled Stuffed - Steak	1	680	28	37	8	3	55	1990	77	7	31	5 starch, 2 medium-fat meat, 3 fat
Supreme - Beef	1	440	18	36	8	2	40	1330	52	5	17	3 1/2 starch, 1 medium-fat meat, 2 fat
Supreme - Chicken	1	410	14	30	6	2	45	1270	50	5	21	3 1/2 starch, 1 medium-fat meat, 1 fat

Supreme - Steak	1	420	16	34	7	2	35	1260	50	6	19	3 1/2 starch, 1 medium-fat meat, 1 1/2 fat

CHALUPAS

Baja - Beef	1	430	28	58	7	2	30	760	32	2	13	2 starch, 1 medium-fat meat, 4 1/2 fat
Baja - Chicken	1	400	24	54	5	2	40	710	30	2	17	2 starch, 1 medium-fat meat, 1 1/2 fat
Baja - Steak	1	410	25	54	6	2	30	700	30	2	15	2 starch, 1 medium-fat meat, 3 1/2 fat
Nacho Cheese - Beef	1	380	22	52	5	3	20	760	33	2	12	2 starch, 1 medium-fat meat, 3 1/2 fat
✔Nacho Cheese - Chicken	1	350	18	46	4	3	25	700	31	2	16	2 starch, 2 medium-fat meat, 1 fat
✔Nacho Cheese - Steak	1	360	20	50	4.5	3	20	690	31	2	14	2 starch, 1 medium-fat meat, 2 1/2 fat

(Continued)

✔ = Healthiest Bets

CHALUPAS *(Continued)*	Amount	Cal.	Fat (g)	% Cal. Fat	Sat. Fat (g)	Trans Fat (g)	Chol. (mg)	Sod. (mg)	Carb. (g)	Fiber (g)	Pro. (g)	Servings/Exchanges
Supreme - Beef	1	400	24	54	8	2.5	35	600	31	1	14	2 starch, 1 medium-fat meat, 3 1/2 fat
✔Supreme - Chicken	1	370	21	51	7	2	45	530	29	2	17	2 starch, 1 medium-fat meat, 3 fat
Supreme - Steak	1	370	22	53	7	2	35	550	29	2	15	2 starch, 1 medium-fat meat, 3 1/2 fat
EXPRESS MENU ITEMS												
Express Taco Salad	1	610	30	44	12	2.5	65	1440	61	10	26	4 starch, 2 medium-fat meat, 3 1/2 fat
Grilled Stuffed Burrito - Beef	1	720	32	40	11	3	55	2120	81	7	27	5 starch, 2 medium-fat meat, 4 fat
Grilled Stuffed Burrito - Chicken	1	670	24	32	7	2.5	70	1990	78	7	35	5 starch, 3 medium-fat meat, 1 1/2 fat

Grilled Stuffed Burrito - Steak	1	670	27	36	8	3	55	1970	77	7	31	5 starch, 2 medium-fat meat, 3 fat
Nachos	1	310	16	46	3.5	3	4	580	36	2	5	2 starch, 3 fat
Nachos Bell Grande	1	750	36	43	10	5	35	1400	86	10	20	5 1/2 starch, 1 medium-fat meat, 5 fat
Nachos Supreme	1	440	22	45	8	3	30	860	45	5	13	3 starch, 1 high-fat meat, 2 1/2 fat
Southwest Steak Border Bowl	1	660	25	34	9	2.5	55	2230	81	10	30	5 starch, 2 medium-fat meat, 2 1/2 fat
Zesty Chicken Border Bowl	1	710	38	48	8	2.5	45	1760	70	10	23	4 1/2 starch, 1 medium-fat meat, 6 fat
✔Zesty Chicken Border Bowl w/out dressing	1	470	14	26	4.5	2.5	30	151	65	1	22	4 starch, 1 medium-fat meat, 2 fat

FRESCO STYLE ITEMS

✔Tostada	1	200	6	27	1	1	0	670	30	8	8	2 starch, 1 1/2 fat

✔ = Healthiest Bets

(Continued)

	Amount	Cal.	Fat (g)	% Cal. Fat	Sat. Fat (g)	Trans Fat (g)	Chol. (mg)	Sod. (mg)	Carb. (g)	Fiber (g)	Pro. (g)	Servings/Exchanges
FRESCO STYLE ITEMS – BURRITO												
Bean	1	350	8	20	2	2	0	1220	56	9	13	3 1/2 starch, 1 1/2 fat
Fiesta - Chicken	1	340	8	21	2	1.5	25	1160	50	3	16	3 starch, 1 medium-fat meat, 1/2 fat
Supreme - Chicken	1	350	8	20	2	1.5	25	1270	50	6	19	3 1/2 starch, 1 medium-fat meat
Supreme - Steak	1	350	9	23	2.5	1.5	15	1260	50	6	17	3 1/2 starch, 1 medium-fat meat
FRESCO STYLE ITEMS – ENCHIRITO												
Beef	1	270	9	30	3	1	20	1300	35	5	12	2 starch, 1 medium-fat meat, 1 fat
Chicken	1	250	5	18	1.5	1	25	1230	34	5	16	2 starch, 1 medium-fat meat

Steak	1	250	7	25	2	1	15	1220	34	3	14	2 starch, 1 medium-fat meat

FRESCO STYLE ITEMS – GORDITA BAJA

✔Beef	1	250	9	32	3	0	20	640	31	2	12	2 starch, 1 medium-fat meat
✔Chicken	1	230	6	23	1	0	25	570	29	2	15	2 starch, 1 medium-fat meat
✔Steak	1	230	7	27	1.5	0	15	570	29	3	13	2 starch, 1 medium-fat meat

FRESCO STYLE ITEMS – TACO

✔Crunchy	1	150	7	42	2.5	0.5	20	360	14	2	7	1 starch, 1 1/2 fat
✔Grilled Steak Soft	1	170	5	26	1.5	0.5	15	560	21	2	11	1 1/2 starch, 1 fat
✔Ranchero Chicken Soft	1	170	4	21	1	0.5	25	710	22	2	12	1 1/2 starch, 1 fat
✔Soft – Beef	1	190	8	37	2.5	1	20	630	22	2	9	1 1/2 starch, 1 1/2 fat

✔ = Healthiest Bets

(Continued)

	Amount	Cal.	Fat (g)	% Cal. Fat	Sat. Fat (g)	Trans Fat (g)	Chol. (mg)	Sod. (mg)	Carb. (g)	Fiber (g)	Pro. (g)	Servings/Exchanges
GORDITAS - BAJA												
✔Beef	1	350	19	48	5	0.5	30	760	31	2	13	2 starch, 1 medium-fat meat, 2 1/2 fat
✔Chicken	1	320	15	42	3.5	0	40	690	29	2	17	2 starch, 1 medium-fat meat, 2 fat
✔Steak	1	320	16	45	4	0	30	680	29	2	15	2 starch, 1 medium-fat meat, 2 fat
GORDITAS - NACHO CHEESE												
✔Beef	1	300	13	39	4	1.5	20	740	32	2	12	2 starch, 1 medium-fat meat, 1 1/2 fat
✔Chicken	1	270	10	33	2.5	1	25	670	30	2	16	2 starch, 1 medium-fat meat, 1/2 fat
✔Steak	1	270	11	36	3	1.5	20	660	30	2	14	2 starch, 1 high-fat meat, 1/2 fat

GORDITAS - SUPREME

	Amount										
✔ Beef	1	310	16	46	7	0.5	35	600	30	2	14	2 starch, 1 high-fat meat, 1 1/2 fat
✔ Chicken	1	290	12	37	5	0	45	530	28	2	17	2 starch, 1 high-fat meat, 1 fat
✔ Steak	1	290	13	40	6	0.5	35	520	28	2	16	2 starch, 1 medium-fat meat, 1 1/2 fat

NACHOS

Nachos	1	320	19	53	4.5	4	4	530	33	2	4	2 starch, 4 fat
Nachos Bell Grande	1	790	44	50	12	7	35	1300	79	10	19	5 starch, 8 1/2 fat
Nachos Supreme	1	460	26	50	8	3.5	35	810	42	5	13	3 starch, 5 fat

SIDES

✔ Cinnamon Twists	1	160	5	28	1	1	0	220	27	0	1	2 starch, 1/2 fat
Mexican Rice	1	200	9	40	3.5	0.5	15	850	26	2	3	1 1/2 starch, 2 fat

(Continued)

✔ = Healthiest Bets

SIDES *(Continued)*	Amount	Cal.	Fat (g)	% Cal. Fat	Sat. Fat (g)	Trans Fat (g)	Chol. (mg)	Sod. (mg)	Carb. (g)	Fiber (g)	Pro. (g)	Servings/Exchanges
Pintos 'n Cheese	1	180	7	35	3.5	1	15	700	20	6	10	1 starch, 1 high-fat meat
SPECIALTIES												
Cheese Quesadilla	1	490	28	51	13	2	55	1150	39	3	19	2 1/2 starch, 2 high-fat meat, 2 fat
Chicken Quesadilla	1	540	30	50	13	2	80	1380	40	3	28	2 1/2 starch, 3 medium-fat meat, 3 fat
Enchirito - Beef	1	380	18	42	9	1.5	45	1430	35	5	19	2 starch, 2 medium-fat meat, 1 fat
Enchirito - Chicken	1	350	14	36	7	1.5	55	1360	33	5	23	2 starch, 2 medium-fat meat, 1 fat
Enchirito - Steak	1	360	16	40	8	1.5	45	1350	33	5	21	2 starch, 2 medium-fat meat, 1 fat

Express Taco Salad	1	630	34	48	12	3.5	65	1390	58	10	26	3 starch, 3 veg, 2 high-fat meat, 3 fat
Express Taco Salad w/out chips	1	410	21	46	10	1.5	65	1300	32	8	12	1/2 starch, 3 veg, 1 high-fat meat, 4 fat
Fiesta Taco Salad	1	860	46	48	14	5	65	1800	82	12	31	4 1/2 starch, 2 veg, 2 high-fat meat, 6 fat
Fiesta Taco Salad w/ chips	1	630	33	47	13	3.5	65	1390	58	10	26	3 starch, 2 veg, 2 high-fat meat, 3 1/2 fat
Fiesta Taco Salad w/out shell	1	490	25	45	11	2	65	1530	43	10	24	2 starch, 2 veg, 2 high-fat meat, 2 fat
Fiesta Taco Salad w/out shell or red strips	1	420	21	45	10	1.5	65	1480	34	9	24	1/2 starch, 3 veg, 2 high-fat meat, 1 1/2 fat
Mexican Pizza	1	550	31	50	10	3.5	45	1040	47	5	20	3 starch, 2 high-fat meat, 2 1/2 fat
✔Meximelt	1	290	16	49	8	1	40	880	23	2	15	1 1/2 starch, 1 high-fat meat, 1 1/2 fat

✔ = Healthiest Bets

(Continued)

SPECIALTIES *(Continued)*	Amount	Cal.	Fat (g)	% Cal. Fat	Sat. Fat (g)	Trans Fat (g)	Chol. (mg)	Sod. (mg)	Carb. (g)	Fiber (g)	Pro. (g)	Servings/Exchanges
Southwest Steak Bowl	1	690	28	36	8	2.5	55	2330	79	10	30	5 starch, 2 medium-fat meat, 4 fat
Steak Quesadilla	1	540	31	51	14	2	70	1370	40	3	26	2 1/2 starch, 3 medium-fat meat, 2 fat
✔Tostada	1	250	10	36	4	1.5	15	710	29	7	11	2 starch, 1 high-fat meat
Zesty Chicken Border Bowl	1	730	40	49	8	2.5	45	1810	69	10	23	3 1/2 starch, 3 veg, 2 medium-fat meat, 3 fat
Zesty Chicken Border Bowl w/out dressing	1	490	16	29	4	2.5	30	1570	64	10	22	3 starch, 3 veg, 2 medium-fat meat, 1 fat
TACOS												
✔Crunchy	1	170	10	52	4	0.5	25	350	13	0	8	1 starch, 1 high-fat meat

Item											Exchanges
✔ Double Decker Supreme	1	380	18	42	8	2	40	820	41	5	15	3 starch, 1 high-fat meat, 1 1/2 fat
✔ Grilled Steak Soft	1	280	17	54	4.5	1	30	650	21	1	12	1 1/2 starch, 1 medium-fat meat, 2 fat
✔ Ranchero Chicken Soft Taco	1	270	14	46	4	0.5	35	710	21	1	14	1 1/2 starch, 1 medium-fat meat, 1 1/2 fat
✔ Soft - Beef	1	210	10	42	4	1	25	620	21	0	10	1 1/2 starch, 1 medium-fat meat, 1/2 fat
✔ Soft Supreme - Beef	1	260	14	48	7	1	35	640	23	1	11	1 1/2 starch, 1 medium-fat meat, 1/2 fat
✔ Supreme	1	220	14	57	7	1	35	360	14	1	9	1 starch, 1 high-fat meat, 1 fat

✔ = Healthiest Bets

Wendy's

www.wendys.com

Light & Lean Choice

**1 Mandarin Chicken Salad with
Roasted Almonds (1 packet)
Low-Fat Honey Mustard Dressing
(2 T or 1/2 packet)
1 Frosty Jr.**

Calories	515	Cholesterol (mg)	75
Fat (g)	18	Sodium (mg)	795
% calories from fat	31	Carbohydrate (g)	60
Saturated fat (g)	4	Fiber (g)	5
Trans fat (g)	0	Protein (g)	32

Exchanges: 2 carb, 2 vegetable, 3 lean meat, 2 fat

Healthy & Hearty Choice

**1 Baked Potato (plain)
1 Chili (large bowl)
1 Side Salad
Reduced-Fat Cream Ranch Dressing
(2 T or 1/2 packet)**

Calories	685	Cholesterol (mg)	62
Fat (g)	13	Sodium (mg)	1,490
% calories from fat	17	Carbohydrate (g)	106
Saturated fat (g)	4	Fiber (g)	19
Trans fat (g)	1	Protein (g)	35

Exchanges: 7 starch, 1 vegetable, 2 medium-fat meat, 1 fat

(*Continued*)

Wendy's

	Amount	Cal.	Fat (g)	% Cal. Fat	Sat. Fat (g)	Trans Fat (g)	Chol. (mg)	Sod. (mg)	Carb. (g)	Fiber (g)	Pro. (g)	Servings/Exchanges
BAKED POTATOES												
✔ Bacon and Cheese	1	460	13	25	5	0	40	740	69	8	16	4 1/2 starch, 1 medium-fat meat, 1 fat
✔ Broccoli and Cheese	1	340	3.5	9	1	0	10	430	69	9	10	4 1/2 starch, 1/2 fat
✔ Plain	1	270	0	0	0	0	0	25	61	7	7	4 starch
✔ Sour Cream and Chives	1	320	4	11	2	0	10	55	63	7	9	4 starch, 1 fat
CHICKEN STRIPS AND NUGGETS												
✔ Chicken Nuggets	5 pc.	220	14	57	3	1.5	35	490	13	0	10	1 starch, 1 medium-fat meat, 2 fat
✔ Chicken Nuggets Kids' Meal	4 pc.	180	11	55	2.5	1.5	25	390	10	0	8	1/2 starch, 1 medium-fat meat, 1 fat

	Amount	Cal.	Fat (g)	% Cal. Fat	Sat. Fat (g)	Trans Fat (g)	Chol. (mg)	Sod. (mg)	Carb. (g)	Fiber (g)	Pro. (g)	Choices/Exchanges
Homestyle Chicken Strips	3 ea.	410	18	39	3.5	3	60	1470	33	0	28	2 starch, 3 lean meat, 2 fat

CHILI AND FIXINGS

	Amount	Cal.	Fat (g)	% Cal. Fat	Sat. Fat (g)	Trans Fat (g)	Chol. (mg)	Sod. (mg)	Carb. (g)	Fiber (g)	Pro. (g)	Choices/Exchanges
✔ Cheddar Cheese, shredded	2 T	70	6	77	3.5	0	15	110	1	0	4	1 medium-fat meat
Large Chili	1	330	9	24	3.5	0.5	55	1170	35	8	25	2 starch, 3 lean meat
✔ Saltine Crackers	2 ea.	25	0.5	18	0	0	0	95	4	0	1	1/2 starch
✔ Small Chili	1	220	6	24	2.5	0	35	780	23	5	17	1 1/2 starch, 2 lean meat

FRIES

	Amount	Cal.	Fat (g)	% Cal. Fat	Sat. Fat (g)	Trans Fat (g)	Chol. (mg)	Sod. (mg)	Carb. (g)	Fiber (g)	Pro. (g)	Choices/Exchanges
Biggie	5.6 oz	490	24	44	4	6	0	480	64	6	5	4 starch, 4 fat
Great Biggie	6.7 oz	590	28	42	5	7	0	570	77	7	6	5 starch, 4 1/2 fat
Kids' Meal	3.2 oz	280	14	45	2.5	3.5	0	270	37	3	3	2 starch, 2 fat
Medium	5.0 oz	440	21	42	3.5	5	0	430	58	5	5	4 starch, 3 fat

(Continued)

✔ = Healthiest Bets

	Amount	Cal.	Fat (g)	% Cal. Fat	Sat. Fat (g)	Trans Fat (g)	Chol. (mg)	Sod. (mg)	Carb. (g)	Fiber (g)	Pro. (g)	Servings/Exchanges
FROSTY												
✔Fix 'n Mix Frosty	1	170	4	21	2.5	0	20	80	29	0	4	2 carb, 1/2 fat
✔Frosty Junior	6 oz	160	4	22	2.5	0	15	75	28	0	4	2 carb, 1/2 fat
Frosty Medium	16 oz	430	11	23	7	0	45	200	74	0	10	5 carb, 2 fat
Frosty Small	12 oz	330	8	21	5	0	35	150	56	0	8	3 1/2 carb, 1 1/2 fat
Frosty Mix-ins												
Butterfinger Candy Crumbles	1 pkt.	130	5	34	2.5	0	0	65	20	1	2	1 carb, 1 fat
M&M's Candy Crumbles	1 pkt.	140	6	38	3.5	0	5	15	20	1	1	1 carb, 1 1/2 fat
Oreo Cookie Crumbles	1 pkt.	100	4.5	40	1	1.5	0	110	15	1	1	1 carb, 1 fat
SALADS/SIDES												
✔Caesar Side Salad	1	70	5	64	2	0	15	135	3	2	5	1 veg, 1 fat

												Exchanges/Choices
✔Chicken BLT	1	340	18	47	9	0	105	840	12	4	34	1 starch, 4 lean meat, 1 fat
Homestyle Chicken Strips	1	450	22	44	8	2.5	70	1190	35	4	29	1 1/2 starch, 2 veg, 3 medium-fat meat, 1 fat
✔Low-Fat Strawberry Flavored Yogurt	1	200	2	9	1	0	10	120	37	0	8	1 1/2 carb, 1 milk
✔Mandarin Chicken	1	170	2	10	0.5	0	60	480	18	3	23	1/2 starch, 2 veg, 2 very-lean meat
✔Mandarin Orange Cup	1	80	0	0	0	0	0	15	19	1	1	1 fruit
✔Side Salad	1	35	0	0	0	0	0	20	7	3	2	1 veg
✔Spring Mix	1	180	11	55	6	0	30	230	13	4	10	2 veg, 1 medium-fat meat, 1 fat
✔Taco Supremo	1	380	17	40	9	0.5	65	1000	33	9	27	1 1/2 starch, 2 veg, 2 high-fat meat

(Continued)

✔ = Healthiest Bets

	Amount	Cal.	Fat (g)	% Cal. Fat	Sat. Fat (g)	Trans Fat (g)	Chol. (mg)	Sod. (mg)	Carb. (g)	Fiber (g)	Pro. (g)	Servings/Exchanges
SANDWICHES												
Big Bacon Classic	1	580	29	45	12	1.5	95	1400	46	3	35	3 starch, 3 high-fat meat, 1 fat
✔Cheeseburger Kids' Meal	1	320	13	36	6	0.5	40	820	34	1	17	2 starch, 2 medium-fat meat, 1/2 fat
✔Classic Single w/ Everything	1	420	19	40	7	1	65	900	37	2	25	2 1/2 starch, 2 medium-fat meat, 1 1/2 fat
✔Hamburger Kids' Meal	1	270	9	30	3.5	0.5	30	600	33	1	15	2 starch, 1 medium-fat meat, 1 1/2 fat
Homestyle Chicken Fillet	1	540	22	36	4	1.5	55	1350	57	2	29	3 1/2 starch, 2 medium-fat meat, 2 fat
✔Jr. Bacon Cheeseburger	1	380	18	42	7	0.5	55	810	34	2	20	2 starch, 2 medium-fat meat, 1 fat

✔ Jr. Cheeseburger	1	320	13	36	6	0.5	40	820	34	1	17	2 starch, 1 medium-fat meat, 1 1/2 fat
✔ Jr. Cheeseburger Deluxe	1	360	15	37	6	0.5	45	880	37	2	18	2 starch, 2 medium-fat meat, 2 fat
✔ Jr. Hamburger	1	280	9	28	3.5	0.5	30	600	34	1	15	2 starch, 1 medium-fat meat, 1/2 fat
Spicy Chicken Fillet Sandwich	1	510	18	31	3.5	1.5	55	1470	57	2	29	4 starch, 2 medium-fat meat, 1 fat
Ultimate Grilled Chicken Sandwich	1	360	7	17	1.5	0	75	1100	44	2	31	3 starch, 2 lean meat

TOPPINGS AND DRESSINGS

✔ Barbecue Sauce	1 pkt/4 T	40	0	0	0	0	0	160	10	0	1	1/2 carb
✔ Caesar Dressing	1 pkt/4 T	120	13	97	2.5	0	20	220	1	0	1	3 fat
Creamy Ranch Dressing	1 pkt/4 T	230	23	90	4	0	15	450	5	0	1	5 fat

✔ = Healthiest Bets

(Continued)

TOPPINGS AND DRESSINGS (Continued)	Amount	Cal.	Fat (g)	% Cal. Fat	Sat. Fat (g)	Trans Fat (g)	Chol. (mg)	Sod. (mg)	Carb. (g)	Fiber (g)	Pro. (g)	Servings/Exchanges
✔ Crispy Noodles	1 pkt.	60	2	30	0	0.5	0	170	10	0	1	1/2 starch
Deli Honey Mustard Sauce	1 pkt.	170	16	84	2.5	0	15	190	6	0	0	1/2 carb, 3 fat
✔ Fat Free French Style Dressing	1 pkt/4 T	80	0	0	0	0	0	210	19	0	0	1 carb
✔ Heartland Ranch Sauce	1 pkt/4 T	200	22	99	3.5	0	15	280	1	0	0	4 fat
✔ Homestyle Garlic Croutons	1 pkt	70	3	38	0	0	0	125	9	0	2	1/2 starch, 1/2 fat
Honey Mustard Dressing	1 pkt/4 T	280	26	83	4	0	25	370	11	0	1	1 carb, 5 fat
✔ Honey Mustard Sauce	1 pkt/4 T	130	12	83	2	0	10	220	6	0	0	1/2 carb, 2 fat
✔ House Vinaigrette Dressing	1 pkt/4 T	190	18	85	2.5	0	0	740	8	0	0	1/2 carb, 3 fat
✔ Low Fat Honey Mustard Dressing	1 pkt/4 T	110	3	24	0	0	0	340	21	0	0	1 1/2 carb
✔ Oriental Sesame Dressing	1 pkt/4 T	190	11	52	1.5	0	0	490	21	0	1	1 carb, 2 fat

	Amount										
✔Reduced Fat Creamy Ranch Dressing	1 pkt/4 T	100	8	72	1.5	0	15	450	6	1	1	2 fat
✔Reduced Fat Sour Cream	2 T	50	4	72	2	0	10	30	2	0	1	1 fat
✔Roasted Almonds	1 pkt	130	11	76	1	0	0	70	4	2	5	2 1/2 fat
✔Salsa	1 pkt	30	0	0	0	0	0	440	6	1	1	1 veg
Spicy Southwest Chipotle Sauce	2 T	150	15	90	2.5	0	25	180	5	0	1	3 fat
✔Sweet and Sour Sauce	2 T	50	0	0	0	0	0	120	12	0	0	1 carb
Taco Chips	1 pkt	210	9	38	1	0	0	230	29	2	3	2 starch, 2 fat

✔ = Healthiest Bets

Other Books by Hope Warshaw
from the American Diabetes Association

Diabetes Meal Planning Made Easy, 3rd edition

Hope Warshaw, MMSc, RD, CDE, BC-ADM

Meal planning doesn't have to be complicated. This book will help you simplify your life--and eat healthier meals--by teaching you how to:

- ◆ easily add more fruits and vegetables to your meal plan
- ◆ avoid unhealthy fats
- ◆ make healthy food choices when you're away from home.

292 pages, softcover. ◆ #4706-03 ◆ One low price: $14.95

Complete Guide to Carb Counting, 2nd edition

Hope S. Warshaw, MMSc, RD, CDE, BC-ADM, and
Karmeen Kulkarni, MS, RD, CDE

Learn how to count carbs easily and effortlessly for improved blood sugar control, effective weight loss, and proper nutrition. End the confusion of how to count, what counts, and how much counts with the tools and techniques in this newly updated edition. Even if you purchased the earlier edition, this book is a must-have because it begins where the previous one left off. New chapters include:

- ◆ carb counting for insulin pump users
- ◆ a whole week of meal plans
- ◆ and much more.

262 pages, softcover. ◆ #4715-02 ◆ Nonmember: $16.95 Member: $14.95

The Diabetes Food and Nutrition Bible

Hope S. Warshaw, MMSc, RD, CDE, BC-ADM, and
Robyn Webb, MS

Get the nutrition advice you need and the flavor-rich recipes you crave. Learn about foods that can protect and heal, and get scrumptious recipes to work into your eating plan.

What you learn can have a dramatic effect on the way you eat, what you eat, and how long you live.

325 pages, softcover. ◆ #4714-01 Nonmember: $18.95 Member: $16.95

**Order online at http://store.diabetes.org
or call toll-free at 1-800-232-6733.**

About the American Diabetes Association

The American Diabetes Association is the nation's leading voluntary health organization supporting diabetes research, information, and advocacy. Its mission is to prevent and cure diabetes and to improve the lives of all people affected by diabetes. The American Diabetes Association is the leading publisher of comprehensive diabetes information. Its huge library of practical and authoritative books for people with diabetes covers every aspect of self-care—cooking and nutrition, fitness, weight control, medications, complications, emotional issues, and general self-care.

To order American Diabetes Association books: Call 1-800-232-6733 or log on to http://store.diabetes.org

To join the American Diabetes Association: Call 1-800-806-7801 or log on to www.diabetes.org/membership

For more information about diabetes or ADA programs and services: Call 1-800-342-2383. E-mail: AskADA@diabetes.org or log on to www.diabetes.org

To locate an ADA/NCQA Recognized Provider of quality diabetes care in your area: www.ncqa.org/dprp

To find an ADA Recognized Education Program in your area: Call 1-800-342-2383. www.diabetes.org/for-health-professionals-and-scientists/recognition/edrecognition.jsp

To join the fight to increase funding for diabetes research, end discrimination, and improve insurance coverage: Call 1-800-342-2383. www.diabetes.org/advocacy-and-legalresources/advocacy.jsp

To find out how you can get involved with the programs in your community: Call 1-800-342-2383. See below for program Web addresses.

- *American Diabetes Month:* educational activities aimed at those diagnosed with diabetes—month of November. www.diabetes.org/communityprograms-and-localevents/americandiabetesmonth.jsp
- *American Diabetes Alert:* annual public awareness campaign to find the undiagnosed—held the fourth Tuesday in March. www.diabetes.org/communityprograms-and-localevents/americandiabetesalert.jsp
- *The Diabetes Assistance & Resources Program (DAR):* diabetes awareness program targeted to the Latino community. www.diabetes.org/communityprograms-and-localevents/latinos.jsp
- *African American Program:* diabetes awareness program targeted to the African American community. www.diabetes.org/communityprograms-and-localevents/africanamericans.jsp
- *Awakening the Spirit: Pathways to Diabetes Prevention & Control:* diabetes awareness program targeted to the Native American community. www.diabetes.org/communityprograms-and-localevents/nativeamericans.jsp

To find out about an important research project regarding type 2 diabetes: www.diabetes.org/diabetes-research/research-home.jsp

To obtain information on making a planned gift or charitable bequest: Call 1-888-700-7029. www.wpg.cc/stl/CDA/homepage/1,1006,509,00.html

To make a donation or memorial contribution: Call 1-800-342-2383. www.diabetes.org/support-the-cause/make-a-donation.jsp